Now I Lay
Me Down

The Owner's Manual For The Dying Patient, Their Caregivers and Their Loved Ones

By

Constance Hope Stringer, R.N.

authorHOUSE™

1663 LIBERTY DRIVE, SUITE 200
BLOOMINGTON, INDIANA 47403
(800) 839-8640
WWW.AUTHORHOUSE.COM

© 2005 Constance Hope Stringer, R.N. All Rights Reserved.

No part of this book may be reproduced, stored in a retrieval system, or transmitted by any means without the written permission of the author.

First published by AuthorHouse 07/05/05

ISBN: 1-4208-5223-X (sc)
ISBN: 1-4208-5226-4 (hc)

Printed in the United States of America
Bloomington, Indiana

This book is printed on acid-free paper.

TABLE OF CONTENTS

18TH CENTURY CHILD'S BEDTIME PRAYER:

Now I lay me down to sleep,
I pray the Lord my soul to keep.
If I should die before I wake,
I pray the Lord my soul to take.

DERIVED FROM AN OLD ENGLISH PRAYER:

Matthew, Mark, Luke and John
bless the bed that I lie on.
Before I lay me down to sleep,
I give my soul to Christ to keep.
Four corners to my bed,
four angels there aspread,
two to foot, and two to head,
and two to carry me when I'm dead.
I go by sea, I go by land,
the Lord made me by his right hand.
If any danger comes to me,
sweet Jesus Christ deliver me.
He's the branch, and I'm the flower,
Pray God send me a happy hour.
And if I die before I wake,
I pray that Christ my soul will take.

unknown author

A RIDDLE

What is greater than God?

Worse than the Devil?

Rich people want it.

Poor people have it.

If you eat it you will die!

(Find the answer after reading this book.)

INTRODUCTION

This manual is intended to provide assistance to the dying and their loved ones. This difficult task begins from the moment that a person learns that they, or a loved one, has a terminal illness. For the dying patient it ends with their death, but for the loved ones left behind the grief, bereavement, and mourning sometimes lasts until the day that they, themselves, die.

A "good death" of a loved one helps to improve the quality of life left to those dying, and of those left behind. This book will assist all involved to ensure that the dying person, as well as their loved ones, are adequately cared for physically, emotionally and spiritually.

In the back of the book you will find a "maintanence log". It has forms to keep a record of the activities of the day to ensure a smooth transition from caregiver to caregiver. One example is the form used to document pain medications, their dosages and the times they were administered. Keeping accurate records will not only allow caregivers in the home to know when a medication is due, but they will aid in determining if the drug and dosage are adequate for pain control. Please keep it in a designated place to ensure that all parties involved have access to them.

Please accept my sincere condolances and allow me to assist you as best I can by keeping an open mind when reading the contents of this book carefully, and remembering that avoidance of the facts will not make them go away. You must be honest with yourself and those involved in order to make the best of these trying times. Education is the key. Learn all you can, then apply that knowledge in your own special way.

In order to avoid repetition of he/she, him/her, and his/hers throughout the book, I chose the format of a male patient with his wife as his primary caregiver. The information herein applies to those of all ages and both sexes.

PSALM 23

The Lord is my shephard; I shall not want (for anything).
He maketh me to lie down in green pastures:
He leadeth me beside the still waters.

He restoreth my soul:
He leadeth me in the paths of righteousness for His name
sake.

Yea, though I walk through the valley of the shadow of death,
I will fear no evil: for Thou art with me;
Thy rod and Thy staff they comfort me.

Thou preparest a table before me in the presence of mine
enemies:
Thou anointest my head with oil; my cup runneth over.

Surely goodness and mercy shall follow me all the days of my
life:
And I will dwell in the house of the Lord forever.

Chapter One
WHAT IS DEATH?

Technically, life begins when we draw our first breath and death is the point at which we draw our last, causing an end to all vital functions. But death has many more implications.

Before we can even begin to imagine what it must be like for the terminally ill person who knows that he is going to die, we must seriously consider our own death. As you read the questions below try to answer them. You will soon note that every answer is subjective. Every person will have to search deep within themselves in order to find these answers, because they are all based on our individual belief systems. Most of us have not yet asked ourselves these questions, and fewer yet have the answers. Remember that there are no wrong answers. They are your answers; your beliefs. How well do you know yourself?

When you think of dying, is pain the first thing you think of, is it your greatest fear? How can you be sure that you will suffer as little pain as possible? Would you rather suffer some pain in order to remain conscious of your surroundings and be aware during the days you have left? At what point would you rather "just go off to sleep" as opposed to remaining in pain?

Is death just an eternal slumber, or will you one day "wake up" to another existance? Is there a Heaven and a Hell? Are you afraid to die because you fear the price you will have to pay for your transgressions here on Earth? Could it be that the "worst" of sins requires that you spend eternity burning in the hottest of fires, while lesser sins will lessen the heat and suffering?If you've been "good", will you go to heaven to live among God? Will there be so may people in Heaven that only the purest of souls will be able to get close enough to see him, let alone talk with him? Will your number and severity of sins determine to what extent you will suffer or rejoyce? What is the worst of sins? What sins are unforgiveable? What sins have you committed? What do you have to do to be forgiven of your sins? Must you ask forgiveness of those you have sinned against? Can you make up for them in any way? Is God your final judge, or are you? If you die feeling guilt-free, will you be? Will you be aware of the lives of those you left behind? Will you even know them? Will you have no memory of your life here on Earth? Will those left here on Earth remember you? What will they remember about you? Will your dying cause a financial burden on others? Who? What could you do to prevent it? Is there something you wish you had said to someone? Done for someone? Do you believe there are those who will mourn for you for reasons other than what you could have done for them?

How important is it that others feel that you "died with dignity"? Do you feel that you would lose some of that respect if you cry, or show anger, or show fear? Who do you feel you could talk openly and honestly to about any of these things? Who do you feel would truely listen? Would you like to be involved with picking-out your own casket, making your own funeral arrangements, writing your own eulogy? Who would you trust would follow your last wishes---even if they disagreed? Do you have a durable or medical power of attorney, a living will, or a last will and testament? Where is it? Have you ever taken care of someone that was dying? Did you know they were dying? Did they know? Was it a good experience? A bad one? Do you feel that you were able to help them in any way? Were you afraid you'd do something wrong and do more harm than good? Are you afraid now? What are you most afraid of?

(At the beginning of the maintanence log you will find these questions again with a space for answers. Do not write on these pages unless you are the dying person and do not mind others seeing them. If you are a caregiver, write the answers on a seperate page. It is a good idea to write these answers down now, again when you've finished reading this book, and yet again after your loved one has died.)

2

A GOOD LIFE SHOULD BE REWARDED WITH A GOOD DEATH!

CRITICAL CARE UNIT

As I sit here in this room
Where death has visited many times
I wonder if it has left a trace of itself
to remind us of its' existance

I look from bed to bed and remember the faces
of their not-so-long-ago occupants
I look at the red neon signs with arrows
pointing toward doors that many failed to exit

I remember with shame the times I lost my temper
with anger the times I didn't have the answers
and with sorrow the times that all my training
wasn't enough to heal the wounds that afflicted them

But most of all I remember with joy and pride
the times my touch and soothing word
made them forget their shame
their anger
their sorrow
and their pain
if only for a brief moment

Constance Hope Stringer
1985

Chapter Two
HELP FOR THE TERMINALLY ILL

Your doctor has just told you that the illness you have been struggling with is past the point of medical treatment; that nothing else can be done; that you are going to die.

What are you supposed to say to that? How do you respond? "Ok, doc, thanks for all you've done. Have a nice life! Or, "The Hell you say! I'm going to find me a doctor that knows what he's talking about!"

How about somewhere in between? Like, "I know you wouldn't tell me something like that without being absolutely sure, but can we go over all the tests? Can we talk about this just so that I am sure?"

We'd all like to think that we'd do the latter, but there's no way to know what we would do or say in any situation unless or until it happens to us. Truth be told, most people are shocked into silence when they first get that piece of bad news. They go home and go through the stages of denial, anger, and bargaining before they return in hopes that he had made a huge mistake. "The tests were mixed-up with another persons. Some other poor guy is going to die, not me! Besides, what does that mean that there's nothing else to be done. I'm not dead yet! He did say that I have a few months left. What am I supose to do? Go home and twiddle my thumbs for 3-6 months?"

The above situation may have happened to a loved one. Maybe you even reacted the same way. Or maybe they accepted the inevitable, but you weren't willing to accept it yet.

In any event, it is important to accept the prognosis before you can move on. Do what you have to do, but make it quick, there's lots more to be done besides thumb twiddling. Didn't he say there's only a few months left? Aren't things going to get much worse from here on out.

Now you've accepted the worse news a person could get. It's time to get on with the rest of your life. I wish there was a map I could draw for you to show every little step to take from here on out, but there's not. Every person is different, every circumstance is different. I will attempt, though, to give you some guidelines to follow. You must choose which stage you are in, and what feels right to you.

Right from the start I want to tell you about a wonderful program, called Hospice, that will help you in more ways than I can put into words. I know this because I used to work as a Hospice RN and most of my patients and their family and friends told me just that; "I have no words to say how much you have helped". Most Hospice nurses are accepted into the family and become their life-line. In every other field of nursing we are discouraged from becoming involved, but as a Hospice nurse it is a natural process.

It takes a special kind of person to work with dying people. Some family members start out feeling that the nurse has usurped their place in the patients' life. But they end-up not minding at all that the last person the dying patient, even their spouses and children, ask for , and want at their side in the last minutes of life, is their hospice nurse.

Hospice will ensure that you have all the medications, medical supplies and equipment, and support that you need---free of charge! They will visit you as often as needed and determine any needs you may have, ensure that your pain medications are adequate, and teach any caregiver to do anything they are able and willing to do. They do not take the place of caregivers, they are there to help them help you.

The only criteria there is to become a hospice patient is that your doctor has given you a prognosis of six months or less, that you are no longer seeking life saving measures (radiation or chemotherapy) and that you have a caregiver. They will visit you where ever you live (your house, a friends house, or a nursing home), they will admit you to a hospital for uncontrolled symptoms or to treat a side-effect or condition that would otherwise be treated in the hospital, and they will remain in charge of your care while you are there. They will support your family (related or not) during your care and help them with arrangements after your death. They will be there for months, or even years, after you're gone to help them cope with life without you.

Are you physically able to do some of the things you like doing? Is there anything you always meant to do, but never got around to? Are you financially able to do those things? Decide that now. Live like there is no tomorrow! But remember, most of the really important things in our lives are right around us. And best of all, most of the best things in life are free!

Have you given much thought about who has been there for you all along? Who you know cares for you? Who didn't just come out of the woodwork when they heard your bad news? (Do you get the impression that it was secretly good news to them?) I do not mean to imply that all people that suddenly show up after years of absence have an alterior motive, but I have learned that many people feel this way about some, and are not comfortable having them around. It is important that we have people that we love and trust around us during this time. Confide in someone you trust, and find a way to keep the others away.

Now call that person you wish you had apologized to, and do it.

Call your loved ones to your side and tell them how much they've meant to you; how they've made your life better; give them that piece of advise they'll remember for the rest of their lives (ie: never go to sleep angry).

If you've been angry or upset about something in your life, and there's no way to make it better, let it go. Let go of all of the bad things and hold on to the good!

Time to take care of unfinished business. Balance the checkbook. See were you stand. Transfer funds. Sell that car you've been meaning to sell. Write checks to those you want to have something, if your finances allow, so they won't have to pay inheritence taxes. Tell your wife were the life insurance policy is. Put everything in her name. What ever it takes to get that load off of your shoulders. Take a day or two and think about nothing but this until it is resolved.

Now take out a piece of paper and write down the things you enjoy doing, starting with the things that require the amount of physical activity you are capable of at this point, ending with those that require none. If you are still able to enjoy food, make a list of your favorites. Now, concentrate on the things you enjoy in life. Your frame of mind and attitude about life, and death, is going to determine the course of the rest of your life. Let those who care for you do what they can to improve your quality of life, but remember to be an active participant!

RESTING PEACEFULLY

You lie so still as you sleep
The corners of you mouth turned upward
breathing so quietly, peacefully

As I watch in awe of you
I wonder whos' world you are in
What place could be so heavenly

You seem so far away
So settled, as if to be there for days
So unaware of me

I long to be there with you
The one in your dreams
The cause of that heavenly smile

Then I whisper, "I love you"
Though I know you can not hear
Hoping to somehow touch your world

And you return my love
As you reach out for me in your sleep
And whisper, "I love you, too"

A tear escapes as I realize
You're not in someone else's world
You're resting peacefully in mine!

Constance Hope Stringer
1990

Chapter Three
CARING FOR THE CAREGIVER

Your loved one is dying. Wow, what an awesome responsibility for you! Yes, they are the one that's dying, but what about you? You're losing someone you love! You're losing a financial partner! Your life is about to change drastically, before and after they're gone. AND

You have to decide how best to take care of them! On top of all of this, they are getting all the attention. No one seems to know, or even care, what you are going through. And if that's not enough, you feel selfish for even having that thought!

Well, don't feel guilty. You will be having a lot more thoughts that you will admonish yourself for in the days and months ahead. It's natural. No, we don't go around saying them. We would be quite selfish if we went around demanding that people recognize our sacrifices and loses. But this is a book about honesty. I can't pull any punches if I intend to connect with my readers on important topics. So let me just say it; you are the one I'm most worried about, dear. I hope above all else that your loved one is kept happy and comfortable for the rest of his days, but, let's face it, you're going to need help, too. I know you'll do the right thing and take care of him---you're reading this book aren't you. You'll do all you can to ensure that his last days are happy and comfortable. I'm sorry for his misfortune, but some are not fortunate enough to have someone like you to see to their needs.

Whatever the readers' relationship is to the dying, Thank you for caring enough to not only be there for them, but for wanting to do it right.

The first piece of advise I have for you is to remember that as long as what you do comes from the heart you will do no wrong. With all of the responsibilities you have accepted (cooking, cleaning, bathing, administering medications, wiping a tired brow, kissing away a tear, holding a hand, listening, and being up all hours of the night) there is nothing that you have never done before as a wife, a mother, an aunt, or a sister. There may be some strange apparatus, like a catheter or such that you are not familiar with, but nothing that you can cause harm with.

This is an opportunity for you to shine! Any bit of this that you choose to do is a show of love. I can also tell you that, even though you may not hear it in so many words from your dying loved one, they know it. They will feel it with the smallest of things you do and may not say a word, because sometimes there are just not words to express the extent of our appreciation, and the moment passes without a word rather than chance belittling it with a mear, "Thank you". He'll lay there and bask in your love. What do you think he thinks about all those quiet hours? Watch his face, you'll see.

So, put all those worries out of your mind about wether or not you can care for him the way he deserves to be cared for. He deserves you, and anyone else who is able and willing to help you. Give them the opportunity to help. They want to. There is always room for more help. Even if it is nothing more than sitting at his side reading a book. This brings me back to my point, you. You are the one that's going to need the help. You will need to get out of the house every once in a while. Hopefully you still have your health. Take care of it, you'll need it for him, and for you.

If he is not yet a Hospice patient, and he qualifies, I urge you to contact them. Their social workers are trained in helping people to cope during these trying times. You'd be suprised how much it will help to just talk to someone who understands how you are feeling. There are even scheduled meetings of family members that have been in your place. They even have nurse aides that will do the tasks the patient use to do and is no longer able to. This includes giving their baths! Then get together with friends and family members and decide who is going to do what and when. Write it down. Example: John will mow the lawn on Wednesdays, Susan will cook supper on Mondays, Lisa will stay from noon 'til 3pm on Thursdays, etc. Be flexible when things come up, but let each of them know that you are all counting on eachother. Keep this book in a designated place for all the caregivers to read. If you keep the logs in the back of the book up to date it will help to ensure continuity of care.

LOVE IS FREE

Love is free, love is easy
Don't try to buy me, don't try so hard

Buy me gifts and send me roses
But let them all come from the heart

Touch me gently, kiss me soft
And tell me that you love me so

Think of me when we're not together
But then be sure to let me know!

Constance Hope Stringer
1981

Chapter Four
TROUBLED SEAS

There are five recognized stages of dying. The dying person may not necessarily experience all of them, nor in any particular order. I recently took care of my brother in my home during the last few months of his life. He was only one and a half years older than me when he died of metastatic cancer shortly after he turned 48 years old. He never got out of the denial stage. He continually insisted that he would be going back to work in a matter of days, even when he was too weak to bath himself or go to the toilet. My husband is two weeks older than me. He was very helpfull with my brother's care. He was very patient and kind. Even when my brother began attacking him for doing the very thing my brother asked him to do; take over his job and see to it that the building of structures and other tasks were done correctly. My brother tried to pit me against my husband. He sabbotaged my husband at work by calling up clients and telling lies. It was sad to see someone barely able to talk say such terrible things. He did not belief in God, and was not himself a Godly person. I suspect he was very afraid of dying, but refused to talk about it because he refused to believe he would.

If it had been necessary, we could have dealt with it the two weeks it took for him to die, but thankfully I had a sister that was willing to take him in. He continued to bad mouth my husband and insist that he would get better until the day he died.

I tell you this story to say that, even with the best of intentions, sometimes it is better for all involved, including the dying patient, to be in a different environment. If current arrangements are causing more harm than good, change them. If attempts to help the dying patient through the stages of denial, anger, bargaining and depression, so that they may reach acceptance, are unsuccessfull, then there may be trouble at home. Seek assistance anywhere you can. Weigh the good against the bad and make an informed decision. Do not tough-it-out just to prove that you can. If any aspect of caring for the dying patient becomes too burdensome for you, let someone else take over.

With that said, I sincerely hope for a more pleasant outcome for you.

THE DARK BLUE SEA

Sometimes I feel I'm falling
Far too far to see
I know not where I'm falling
Just in a dark blue sea
People around are talking
They speak no words for me
And people around are walking
But where I can not see
The fall of man I see ahead
I want to stop and scream
But I keep walking on instead
Into life's troubled sea
Look, yonder goes my father
Hey dad, please wait for me
Look, yonder goes my brother
Into the dark blue sea
Ahead there stands a maiden
As fair as one could be
I want to warn this maiden
About the dark blue sea
They kill, they rape, they're saddening
But no one wants to see
The people's tears are adding
Unto the dark blue sea
The flowers hear the wailing
The wind and all the trees
Of people who are sailing
Into life's troubled sea
But can I ever show the world
What life was meant to be
When I am just one lonely pearl
At the bottom of the dark blue sea

Constance Hope Stringer
1974

Chapter Five
CARING FOR THE DYING

Now that you have your support system at the ready, it's time to turn your full attention to matters at hand.

Let's start with the ABC's. The airway is always the number one concern. Is his breathing ok? Does he appear short of breath? If so, ask the doctor or hospice nurse for some oxygen. A concentrator is a machine that takes in the room air and concentrates it. A nasal cannula is a plastic hose that attaches to the concentrator at one end, and wraps around the ears so that the "prongs" where the oxygen excapes rests at the nose. Generally, two liters is adequate to relieve shortness of breath. This is set by turning the knob on the regulator until you see the little ball lift up and the line straight across from the "2" splits the ball in half. If that line is just above the ball it is not quite delivering 2 liters, if the line is below the ball the liter flow is a little over 2 liters.

You will note that the concentrator is a little loud and blows some warm air. Most of my patients preferred to keep the machine in their bedrooms in the fall and winter because of its' heat and soothing "white" noise. In the late spring and summer you may want to keep the machine in another room. Extensions are made to lenghthen the cannula, and the liter flow is accurate up to 50 feet.

Make sure you also have a cannister of oxygen for times that the power may go out, and a small one for travel.

Is there a chance of bleeding, as from a cancerous lesion? If so, make sure there are red or burgandy towels available to absorb it. This will lessen the shock of seeing so much of ones' own (or ones' loved ones') blood. Put them away, out of sight, but remember where they are. They should be cleaned, bagged, and left for this sole purpose.

Are there needles being used for shots of any kind? If so, keep a clorox or milk jug with a secure twist top handy as a sharps container.

Are there narcotics or anti-psycotic drugs being used? If so, keep them out of sight and reach of children and, sad to say, others who may be tempted to abuse them.

Is the patient still able to sit at the dining table? If not, get a bedside or chair-front table. Is his appetite still good, if not ask the doctor or hospice nurse for an appetite stimulant.

Does he experience nausea or vomiting? Get an anti-emetic. If this is a real problem, don't accept pills. How do you keep a pill down when you're throwing-up? You may request that a suppository be used. It will be lubricated and slid as far into the recum as your finger can push it. Or, a nurse can give the medication to him as a shot. If you, or another caregiver, is able and willing, the nurse can teach you how to do this. Emesis basins are not really practical, they're too small and cause a mess. Also, just the sight if one may make him nauseated (power of suggestion). I suggest keeping a small, plastic trash can at his side. It is non-intrusive, cleans-up easily, and can handle the volume and splatters.

Is he past the point of eating? Now, listen up. This is the place that I see family and nurses alike do more harm with good intentions. The body is a miraculous machine. Think of all the things it must do at once, every second of every day. Well, it's more miraculous than most of us know. We experience hunger pains as a way to encourage us to eat when the body needs food, but the dying body literally releases hormones that prevent hunger pains and comforts the dying body in a sense of euphoria! Yes, those who insist on going so far as putting feeding tubes in a dying body are doing them harm. They can't stand the thought of "starving someone to death". If the lack of food is what is killing a person then, by all means, feed that person. But if they are dying from a terminal illness and are either comatose or refusing to eat, respect that and don't force something on them that they do not want nor need.

Does he need a stool softener or laxative? We can't put things in without having something come out. Does he need a bedside commode or bedpan? Diapers, catheter or bedpads?

Does it make him uncomfortable to sleep in a bed with someone else? You need another bed, probably even a hospital bed.

Does he need a shower chair, wheelchair, or walker?

Can you not afford these things, and not have the time or vehicle to go get them? Call hospice. They'll pay for it <u>and</u> bring it to you.

Believe me, I do not own stock in any hospice, nor am I in any way affiliated with one any more. I keep singing its' praises because it is a government funded, non-profit program that is available to anyone that qualifies. The government realized, many years ago, the needs of this special group of people, and developed a specially funded program to ensure that they have all they need during the last six months of their lives. Hospice also accepts donations and has fund raisers so that they can help those in need with things such as the power bill and other necessities during their last days. My greatest disappointment is that so many people die before they have a chance to benefit from it, usually because they either don't know about it, or because the doctors are afraid to tell their patients that no more curative therapy is effective. They are trained to heal and see this as "giving up", or are afraid the patient will see it that way. Please ask your doctor about the program and encourage him to refer you to hospice when the time is right.

And while I'm on that subject, let me tell you that if you must quit your job in order to care for a hospice patient, you may be paid by medicare to do so. It is a necessity to have someone care for those who are dying and can not care for themselves!

You've got the supplies you need, now find a place in the home to store them where they are easily accessable, but unintrusive, This is your home, and should look and feel like one. If you don't have the drawer space for the little things, like diapers, pads, meds, and bedbath supplies, you can get an inexpensive one at Wal-Mart.

If and when he becomes bed-bound, but is still alert enough to enjoy the company of others, you may want to place his bed in the living room (again, hospice can help you with the bed, delivery and the set-up). Do not place the bed in a high traffic area, though; his rest and and privacy are important. You should also consider other aspects of the household (are there small children in the home, etc.), you want to keep him involved in life, but you also have to keep life as normal as possible for others.

Also keep in mind that the smells of cooking may at some point cause him to become nauseated, as well as other smells such as flowers and perfumes. Inform those who wish to send flowers that a green plant would brighten-up his living area, live longer, and not cause respiratory or gastric upset.

If it can be done without clutter, arrange any cards and pictures from loved ones around him. It may be best to get an inexpensive photo album to place them all in and keep at his bedside.

Place a lamp at his bedside, as well as a remote control for the TV or stereo. If you do not have a cordless phone, place a phone at his side, but keep the ringer off.

A room monitor is helpfull (baby monitor). Place the base near him and keep the portable unit with you. This way you won't worry that he needs you when you are busy elsewhere. You can hear every sound he makes.

Have candles and flash lights handy in case of a power outage.

Anticipate his needs and likes. If he is not able to get up and get things for himself, he may choose to do without rather than impose on you. Keep in mind here that sometimes it may appear that he is taking you for granted, and demanding too much of you. Remember that to a person that is inactive, and without much to fill his days, time goes by slowly. What may seem like minutes to you may seem like hours to him. This is not to say that some do not become demanding; some do. In fact, as people go through the stages of denial, anger, bargaining, depression and acceptance, they may be quite demanding. They may even be hateful and hurtful. It is human nature to hurt the ones we love the most, especially if (and because) we are sure of their love for us. Also, some diseases, such as alzheimers', will cause some of these behaviors (see the section on causes of death). Try to understand where they are coming from. If the problem is still too much to handle, seek other arrangements. More than one life is at stake here. The whole idea of caring for a person at home is to ensure a good life, and death.

My moto has always been, "You can say anything, it's how you say it that counts". Find a way to tell them how you feel. It is important to always be honest. Honesty is important in any relationship, but especially to a dying person. They don't want to waste the time they have left playing the silly games most of us play in our daily lives. They need to know that we care enough to set aside the things that don't really matter, and are big enough to face the important things head-on.

All of us have taken care of another person in one capacity or another. You've nursed yourself through colds and illness, and probably many others. Some of you may have read my book "The Owners' Manual For The Body", that details the different systems and functions of the body. For those who haven't, I feel that most of that information is important to know when we are physically taking care of another person, so here it is, a **crash course** in the human body!

MY LOVE, MY LIFE

I look at you and I see
Everything that matters to me
When I think of you I truly feel
That nothing else in life is real

Could it be right to feel this way
Sometimes I wonder what God would say
But He's the one that joined our hearts
I knew that from the very start

The peacefull feeling that it brings
To know that I'm your everything
That you admire and respect me too
Just keeps me longing to please you

That's what makes my life worth living
To know that I'm not only giving
But getting just as much in return
From the man for which my heart does burn

Constance Hope Stringer
2002

Chapter Six
A CRASH COURSE

THE SKIN

Skin is the tissue that covers the surface of the body. The **dermis** is the thick underlayer of connective tissue. There are 5 layers of tissue on the outside of the dermis, called the **epidermis**. The cells of each layer migrate upward as they mature. The epidermis is constantly shedding and reproducing. Modified skin, called **mucous membranes**, lines various parts of the body such as the nose, mouth, vagina, bladder, lungs, and intestines. They are very vascular and capable of absorption of nutrients... and germs.

Our skin holds us together and protects other body systems from the environment. It also helps to control our temperatures by providing the surface for the evaporation of sweat when it's hot and our blood vessels dilate. Our vessels constrict when it's cold, decreasing sweat and conserving heat. In addition to grooming and protecting our skin from bacteria, we must also protect it from injury. The nerves in our skin alert us to dangers to the point of causing pain when we don't respond quickly enough. No pain is natural, it's telling you something, listen to it.

Melanin determines the color of the skin. The more melanin, the deeper the color. Genetic differences determine the amount of melanin in the skin. The UV rays of the sun stimulate the production of melanin, absorbing the rays and darkening the skin.

All skin has a blood supply that keeps it supplied with oxygen and nutrients. Any part of the skin without an adequate blood supply will surely die. Follow the instructions of your nurse and doctor to ensure that this blood supply continues unrestricted. When a person sits or lays for extended periods of time pressure is put onto the skin in some points that closes off the veins and arteries and does not allow blood through. This will cause injury or death to the tissues that are normally supplied by those vessels. Things such as clots also occlude these vessels, as well as some diseases that cause vessels to constrict and severely limit the blood supply, especially to the peripheral circulation (arms/hands and legs/feet).

Some definitions of interest:

• Abrasion: a rubbing away of tissue by friction

• Benign: noncancerous

• Cancer: an uncontrolled, abnormal growth of new tissue

• Cyanosis: a bluish color to the skin caused by not enough oxygen

• Decub (decubitus ulcer): an ulcer caused by pressure

• Dermatitis: inflammation of the skin

• Ischemia: a lack of, or decreased supply of, oxygenated blood to a body part

• Jaundice: a yellow color to the skin caused by too much bilirubin in the blood

• Laceration: cut in tissue

• Malignant: tends to become worse and causes death

• Melanoma: skin cancer

• Metastasis: where tumor cells travel to other parts of the body

• Necrosis: localized tissue death

• Sclerosis: hardening of tissue

• Ulcer: a craterlike wound caused by necrosis of the skin

• Wound: localized injury to tissue

THE SKELETON

The skeleton is the framework of our bodies. It is made-up of 206 bones supporting the adult body. They act to give us form and provide attachments for muscles to allow body movement. The skeleton also provides protection for internal organs. The bones are connected by ligaments and the muscles are connected to the bones by tendons. Bones store and produce red blood cells, platelets, and most white blood cells inside their shafts. This is a spongy substance called the marrow. The skeleton is constantly forming and destructing. Until the age of 35 to 40 years bones are formed faster than they are worn down, after that they destruct faster than they are formed. In advanced age bones become thin and brittle and the vertebrae tend to collapse, actually decreasing the height of the body. More than 90% of the body's calcium is stored in the skeleton. Calcium is an important electrolyte used for the transmission of nerve impulses, muscle contraction, coagulation of the blood, heart function, etc. It is also important for the development and health of your bones.

As a person ages, especially women, more calcium is required in their diet for bone health. It is also important to maintain good posture to ensure proper bone alignment. When a bone is fractured a cast is usually applied.

A cast is a stiff, solid dressing applied to immobilize the limb or body part,during healing. The length of time the cast has to be worn depends on the type or extent of the break and the type of bone that was fractured. Some fractures may require traction. This is another way of immobilizing that limb or body part by applying tension by means of pulleys and weights.

Some definitions of interest:

• Arthritis: inflammation of the joints

• Coccyx: "tail" bone at base of vertebrae

• Femur: long bone in the upper leg

• Fibia: thin, outer bone in lower leg

• Fracture: break in bone

• Humerus: long bone in upper arm

• Kyphosis: convexity in the curvature of the spine (hunchbacked)

• Ligament: fibrous tissue that connects joints, bones, and cartilage

• Mandible: jaw bone

• Myeloma: bone cancer

• Osteoporosis: abnormal loss of bone density (thin bones)

• Osteosarcoma: malignant tumor of bone tissue

• Osteosclerosis: increased density of bone tissue (thickbones)

• Radius: forearm bone on the thumb side

• Sarcoma: bone cancer

• Scoliosis: lateral curvature of the spine (crooked)

• Sternum: long, flat bone in breast/chest

• Tendon: fibrous connective tissue that attaches muscle to bone

• Tibia: large bone in lower leg

• Ulna: forearm bone on "pinky" side

• Vertebrae: back bones

THE MUSCLES

Muscles are a set of fibers or cells that are able to contract. This causes movement. The two basic kinds are striated muscle and smooth muscle. The skeletal muscles are **striated**. They are structured in parallel lines (striped). They are long and respond quickly to stimulation. They are known as voluntary muscles because we can make them move at will. The main muscle of the heart is striated, but it is usually classified as a third kind of muscle, called cardiac muscle, because it is an involuntary muscle.

Smooth muscle is made up of short fibers, giving it a smooth appearance. It composes all the visceral muscles (internal organs). All smooth muscle is involuntary, meaning we do not have conscious control of it (we can't move it at will).

Exercise is an action that is performed repeatedly that causes muscle exertion and serves to maintain or develop strength. It has a beneficial effect on all of the body systems. It is important to exercise often, but if you have health problems ask your doctor what this exercise should consist of. Also, good posture is important to maintain good muscle tone, and good muscle tone helps to protect all of our other body parts.

Some definitions of interest:

• Atrophy: waste away or shrink-up

• Muscle strain: damage from excessive physical effort

• Muscular dystrophy: a group of genetically transmitted diseases characterized by progressive atrophy

• Muscular tone: a normal degree of tension at rest

• Muscular tremor: regular, involuntary contraction

• Myoma: tumor of the uterine muscle

• Tendon: connective tissue that attaches muscle to bone

THE NERVES

A nerve is a fiber that carries impulses, or messages, from the brain to different parts of the body (efferent fibers), or from a part of the body to the brain (afferent fibers). The numerous nerve bundles, or groups of nerves, throughout the body control all of the bodies functions.

The **central nervous system** (CNS) is made up of the brain and spinal cord. It processes information to and from the peripheral nervous system (PNS). Twelve pairs of cranial nerves come directly from the brain. The spinal cord is a long, round cord of 31 pairs of spinal nerves. It is enclosed in 3 layers of protective membranes called the meninges, then surrounded by bones called the vertebrae, or spinal column.

The **peripheral nervous system** is made up of the motor and sensory nerves outside the spinal cord. Injury to a peripheral nerve causes loss of movement and/or feeling to the part of the body it serves. Those nerves that supply the body wall are called somatic nerves, and those supplying the internal organs are called visceral nerves.

The autonomic system are those nerves regulating cardiovascular, respiratory, endocrine, and other involuntary body functions.

When a nerve is damaged it effects the part of the body that it serves. Most people only think of a nerve as something that causes pain. Pain is caused by the nerves sending a message to the brain that there is a danger of injury. The nerves also have the ability to adjust to a constant source and intensity of stimulation so that it takes more stimulation to cause the same reaction. In this way we learn to live with or experience pain different from others. This process is called accommodation. When you go to the doctor or hospital you may frequently be asked if you are in pain, and then to grade your pain. The universal scale for pain is 0-10, 0 meaning that you have no pain at all, and 10 meaning that the pain is worse than you ever imagined. You will be asked to pick a number that best grades your pain. Many patients grade it at 0, when in truth they are experiencing a pain level of 2-3 but have become accustomed to it and do not feel that they will be able to be pain free. Please don't do this. Let us know that your pain is a 2-3, but that it is your acceptable level of pain because in order to be pain free you would require so much medicine that it would alter your level of consciousness. This is common in cancer patients. Please state, "I am at a 2 now, but that is an acceptable level for me". On the other hand, we have many patients that grade their pain level at 10, asking for their pain meds, then follow it up with, "Bring me a cup of coffee and a sandwich and turn on the TV". I believe that either they are afraid they will not have their pain addressed,or they are what we refer to as "drug seekers".

Let me assure you on all accounts:

1) If your pain level is a 10 you will be in tears. I have seen big, grown, stoic men cry openly with pain, and the last thing they would want is a cup of coffee or to watch TV. The system only works when you understand it and use it appropriately.

2) You need not exaggerate in order to get your pain meds. If you state you are having pain and ask for pain meds we will give you whatever the doctor has ordered for you. It is not our place to judge. None of us feels good about giving drugs to people because they are "hooked" on them or want the "high" from them, but even if I truly believe that a patient is not in pain, if they say they are in pain they will get treated for that pain... period. That is the law and, like it or not, we are all required to follow it!

3) Most importantly, if you are in pain, please do not hesitate to let us know! Pain is a serious indicator that something is wrong, and the extent of that pain is an indicator of the extent and seriousness of the problem. Also, pain is a hindrance to your over-all well-being. It is the number one problem that should be addressed, and we feel good when we can do something for you that has such an immediate good response!

Some definitions of interest:

• Anxiety: a feeling of dread or impending danger

• Dementia: progressive deterioration of the mental processes resulting in chronic personality changes, confusion, memory loss and loss of judgement

• Multiple sclerosis (MS): a disease caused by the destruction of the myelin sheath (protective covering of phospholipids and protein) of the brain and spinal cord, causing muscle weakness, poor eyesight, slow speech and inability to move

• Myasthenia Gravis: a condition characterized by chronic muscle weakness and fatigability due to a defect in the conduction of nerve impulses especially in the face and throat causing the person to look slack-faced and droopy-eyed

• Neurological: pertaining to the nervous system

• Neuropathy: inflammation or degeneration of the peripheral nerves

• Paralysis: the loss of muscle function and/or sensation

• Parkinson's disease: slow degeneration of the neurologic system causing a resting tremor, drooling, forwardleaning, shuffling walk, stiff and weak muscles, emotional instability and defective judgement

• Peripheral: the outside, surface, or surrounding area

THE CARDIOVASCULAR SYSTEM

The heart is a cone-shaped, hollow muscular organ, about the size of a man's fist, that sits in the middle of the chest, just slightly to the left. It collects deoxygenated blood from throughout the body and pumps oxygenated blood back to the body at a rate of 60-100 times per minute, when it is functioning properly. The layer on the outside of the heart is called the **epicardium**, the main body is the **myocardium**, and the inner layer is the **endocardium**. The heart is divided into 4 sections, called chambers, by a cross-shaped, thin wall called the septum. The two top chambers are the **atria**, and the two bottom, thick, muscular chambers are the **ventricles**.

When blood enters the heart from the veins, it enters first into the right atrium where it is pushed into the right ventricle, then through a large vessel into smaller vessels lining the lungs where it picks up oxygen and releases carbon dioxide to be exhaled. This oxygen-enriched blood is then pushed into the left atrium, then to the left ventricle where it is forced back into the body's circulation through vessels called **arteries**. Arteries become smaller as they reach the surface layers of skin and muscle and become known as **arterioles**, the smallest of the arteries.

The blood in the arterioles continues on into **capillaries** which are the smallest of the vessels. They are a single cell in thickness, and this is where blood and tissue fluids exchange various substances. Then the blood continues on into **venules**, the smallest of the veins, into **veins** where it travels back into the heart. This system of arteries, arterioles, capillaries, venules, and veins is continuous, forming an unbroken, winding loop.

The **blood pressure** (BP) is most often measured peripherally, with a cuff and regulator called a sphygmomanometer, and is an indirect way of measuring the force of the heartbeat, volume of blood in the body, and the dilatation and constriction of the arteries. The cuff is inflated until the arteries are occluded (closed-off) and no sound can be heard. The pressure is released slowly until a beat can be heard, this is called the systolic blood pressure. The regulator on the sphygmomanometer has a numbered dial with a hand, like on a clock. As air is allowed to escape from the cuff the hand will move along the dial and you will note the number the hand is on when you hear that first sound. This measurement is in millimeters of mercury. As the pressure continues to be released, sounds can be heard until they abruptly disappear or a distinct lessening of these sounds is heard, this is called the diastolic blood pressure.

The normal adult blood pressure is 120/80. A systolic of over 140 or diastolic of over 90 is considered **hypertension**, or high blood pressure. If the BP is high due to stress, emotion, or pain it usually resolves itself quickly. If it is chronic (long standing) it may require medication. Remember that a BP is an indirect way of measuring the volume of blood in the body. This may be due to fluid overload, meaning that you are retaining too much fluid. In this case the doctor may prescribe a diuretic to make you urinate more, therefore decreasing your fluid load. The BP also indirectly measures the constriction of the arteries. If the doctor determines that this is the reason for your hypertension he may prescribe you an antihypertensive. This is a medication that will increase the inner diameter of the arteries, allowing them to hold more volume, therefore decreasing the pressure on them. A systolic of under 100 or diastolic of under 60 is considered **hypotension**, or low blood pressure. We have learned that it is preferable to have a lower pressure than previously thought in the case of heart disease. Trust your doctor and nurse when you are given a medicine that lowers your pressure more than you thought was necessary.

These medicines have multiple beneficial effects in some cases, and is beyond the scope of information I have intended to provide here. In the hospital the doctors set limits on the use of these medications; they tell us at what point to give or withhold a medication. It is always a good idea to ask your doctor the limits for your medications, of any kind. He will tell you the symptoms to watch for and at what point to hold the medicine or to call him for a decision. That being said... Hypotension may be indicative of a low blood volume, as in dehydration or blood loss through bleeding somewhere. This may be treated by administration of IV fluids or a transfusion of blood. It may also be indicative of too much dilatation in the arteries as in too much antihypertensive medication, or too much heat as in "heat stroke". Lay down or sit still for a while, and get out of the sun or sauna. As you may recall, hypotension may also be due to not enough force of the heartbeat, or the heart not beating fast enough. A good rule of thumb is that you are fine unless you are experiencing symptoms. Tell your doctor or nurse if you have dizzy spells, become very weak or fatigued, become pale or sweaty, become nauseated for no apparent reason, have chest pains or palpitations, or just have a funny feeling that you can't explain but feel something is wrong.

The part of the brain that controls involuntary actions of the body constantly sends messages to specialized nodes in the right atrium of the heart initiating an impulse that spreads through other nodes and branches throughout the heart causing it to contract. In a normal heartbeat, both the atria contract at the same time, then the ventricles contract together shortly after the atria. When there is an interference with this normal conduction pathway of electrical impulses the normal rhythm of the heart changes. This can cause numerous abnormalities too technical for my intentions here. Our bodies are very complex and miraculous in the way they can adjust to environmental and emotional changes in order to keep an equilibrium of all systems working together. The heartbeat will increase or decrease in response to emotion, exercise, hormones, temperature, pain, and stress. The normal heart rate is between 60 and 100 beats per minute. You can measure this by placing the tips of your two middle fingers on the thumb side of your wrist. When you feel a pulsing there you are feeling the pressure exerted on those arteries by your heart beating, this is called your **pulse**. Look at a clock or watch with a second hand and count the number of times you feel a pulse in a full minute. This is referred to as your heart rate (HR). (Note: I have included a separate section on blood.)

Some definitions of interest:

• Aneurysm: A dilatation in the wall of a vessel causing a weakness there

• Angina: chest pains caused by a lack of oxygen to the heart muscle from atherosclerosis or spasm of the arteries that supply the heart

• Angioplasty: reconstruction of blood vessels

• Arrhythmia: a deviation from the normal pattern of the heartbeat

• Arteriosclerosis: thickening, calcification, and loss of elasticity of the arteries (hardening of the arteries)

• Atherosclerosis: plaques of cholesterol, lipids and cellular debris on the inside walls of vessels causing a narrowed opening

• Bradycardia: heart rate below 60 beats per minute

• CABG: cardiac artery bypass graft

• CHF (congestive heart failure): where neither ventricle is pumping effectively and less blood goes to the kidneys, making them retain salt and water, increasing the amount of blood the already damaged heart has to pump, making it work even harder. Over time the heart becomes enlarged

• CVA (cerebrovascular accident): a lack of oxygenated blood to a part of the brain caused by occlusion or rupture of the vessel in that part of the brain

• Heart failure: a condition where the heart muscle has been weakened or damaged and can not pump blood properly throughout the body

• Hypertension: systolic blood pressure over 140 or diastolic over 90

• Hypotension: systolic blood pressure under 100 or diastolic under 60

• Left sided heart failure: where the left ventricle is not pumping effectively and blood and fluid back-up into the lungs

• MI (myocardial infarction) aka: heart attack; damage to part of the heart muscle caused by obstruction of the blood flow in an artery that supplies that part of the heart

• Regurgitation: flowing backwards from the normal direction

• Rheumatic disease: an inflammatory disease, caused by a reaction to a special kind of respiratory infection, that may effect the heart, joints, and skin

• Right sided heart failure: where the right ventricle is not pumping effectively and blood and fluid back-up into the general circulation

• Stent: a small rodlike structure used to hold arteries open

• Tachycardia: heart rate over 100 beats per minute

THE LYMPHATIC SYSTEM

As the body has veins for the transportation of blood throughout the body, it has a similar network of vessels to carry the lymph. **Lymph** is the watery fluid, containing leucocytes, erythrocytes, and chyle, originating in the organs and tissues of the body. This system helps to protect and maintain the fluid environment of the whole body by producing, filtering, and carrying lymph and producing various blood cells. The lymph travels through numerous lymph nodes that filter it and produce plasma cells, lymphocytes, and monocytes to fight infection. The lymph also transports fats, proteins, and other substances, and restores 60% of the fluid that filters out of the blood capillaries into the tissues during metabolism. The lymph drains into the blood stream. This system also contains specialized lymphatic organs such as the tonsils, the thymus, and the spleen.

The **thymus** is the primary central gland of the lymphatic system. It is actually two lobes that sit in the mediastinum extending from the bottom of the thyroid gland down to the top of the heart. It produces a hormone, thymosin, critical to the development of the immune system.

The **spleen** is a dark purple, oval-shaped organ that is about 6 inches long by 3 inches wide and 1 inch thick, that sits behind the stomach. It has many functions, but is mainly thought to be for the production, maintenance, storage, and even destruction of red blood cells and platelets. It also produces white blood cells to fight infection. Its size increases during and after digestion, and often during an illness.

Some definitions of interest:

• Bacteria: microorganisms of the Schizomycetes class that causes an infection (a blood, sputum, or urine sample may be taken to test for the specific class, or type, of bacteria so the doctor will know which antibiotic to use to kill it)

• Lymphoma: a type of cancer of the lymphoid tissue, usually malignant. The two main kinds are Hodgkin's disease (mostly young adults) and Non-Hodgkin's Lymphoma, NHL (mostly middle-aged adults). The lymph nodes become enlarged and weakness, fever, weight-loss, and anemia develop. Sometimes the liver and spleen become enlarged, bone lesions develop and malabsorption and gastrointestinal disturbances become severe

• Virus: one of more than 200 parasitic microorganisms that cause infections (antibiotics will not work on a virus, you usually have to let it run its course, getting plenty of rest and fluids so the body can fight it, and treat the symptoms such as cough or fever

THE BLOOD

The main function of the blood is to transport oxygen and other nutrients to the cells and remove waste products, including carbon dioxide. The total volume of blood in the average adult is about 7% to 8% of the body weight. Blood is made-up of a clear yellow fluid, called plasma, and formed elements, called erythrocytes, leucocytes, platelets, and specialized cells.

The formed elements constitute about 50% of the total volume of the blood. The **erythrocytes** are the mature red blood cells, that originate in the bone marrow, that transport oxygen in the blood. Their hemoglobin content is a protein-iron compound that carries oxygen from the lungs to the cells and carbon dioxide from the cells to the lungs. When your hemoglobin content is low it is called anemia. This can be caused by a loss of blood, a decrease in the production of red blood cells, or an increase in the destruction of red blood cells.

The spleen is mainly thought to be for the production, maintenance, storage, and even destruction of red blood cells and platelets. If the body suffers severe hemorrhage (bleeding) the spleen can increase the blood volume by 350ml to 550ml in less than 60 seconds.

The liver is the largest gland in the body, and over 500 functions have been identified. It sits under the right lung in the upper abdomen. 13% of the total blood supply is held in the liver at any given time (1 pint). The liver processes hemoglobin from the iron content. It also converts poisonous ammonia to urea and detoxifies numerous substances (alcohol, nicotine, and other poisons).

The **leucocytes** are the white blood cells that fight infections of bacteria, viruses, and fungi. There are 5 types of leucocytes. Their numbers are often increased with bacterial infections, but not usually with viral infections. The **platelets** are the disc-shaped cells that are essential for the coagulation of blood. They are the smallest cell in the blood. They are formed in the red bone marrow, and some are stored in the spleen. Platelets clump at the site of an injury to a blood vessel within seconds, forming a clot. Other factors are included in forming and maintaining a clot, too indepth for my purpose here.

The **plasma** is the watery portion of blood and lymph. It is made-up of water, electrolytes, fats, proteins, glucose, bilirubin, and gases. It is necessary for the transportation of the formed elements and nutrients. It maintains the acid-base balance of the body, and transports wastes from the tissues. It is essential for the exchange of fluids and electrolytes between the capillaries and the tissues. The plasma cell is involved in fighting infections.

In the event that you require a transfusion of packed red blood cells (PRBC's) or fresh frozen plasma (FFP) you will be required to sign a consent before it begins. You will be given some literature on the subject. Always read the material or ask any questions you may have before signing any consent. This is what is meant by an "informed" consent. I don't say this because a transfusion is dangerous, in fact, it is far less dangerous than many things we do, and the screening for infectious agents is very regulated and thorough.

Some definitions of interest:

• Afebrile: not having a fever

• Anemia: an unacceptable decrease in the level of hemoglobin in the blood

• Coagulation: changing from a liquid into a solid or gelatinous mass

• Embolus: a substance or clot that circulates in the blood stream until it becomes lodged in a vessel

• Febrile: having a fever; body temperature over 98.6 degrees

• Hemophilia: a hereditary bleeding disorder caused by a lack of one of the factors needed for the coagulation of blood

• Leukemia: a group of diseases where there is a large number of immature white blood cells. It is malignant (tends to become worse and to cause death)

• Thrombus: clots of platelets and other elements of the blood attached to the inside of a vein or artery that partially or completely occludes the lumen (opening)

THE RESPIRATORY SYSTEM

The respiratory system is made-up of the organs and structures that perform the exchange of oxygen and carbon dioxide between the air we breathe and the blood circulating through the lungs. It also warms the air we breathe and provides air to pass through the vocal cords for speech. The upper respiratory tract includes the nose and throat, and the lower respiratory tract includes the trachea, bronchus and lungs.

The air enters through the nose or mouth and travels through the trachea, where it branches off into the right and left primary bronchus, which branch off further into secondary bronchi and enters the lungs.

The **lungs** are two highly elastic organs sitting on each side of the chest (thoracic cavity). They are made-up of thousands of little air sacs, called alveoli. The lungs are very vascular, meaning that they have a very good blood supply. When air enters the alveoli the blood in the capillaries "picks up" oxygen molecules from it and "drops off" carbon dioxide to be exhaled. When we are active we naturally take deeper breaths. When we sit or lay we tend to breathe shallow, which only brings fresh air into the alveoli at the top of our lungs. This decreases the surface area of fresh (oxygenated) air coming in contact with the blood supply, therefore decreasing the amount of oxygen molecules that can be "picked-up".

Over a period of time, this can also cause the air sacs at the bottom of our lungs to deflate and makes space for fluid to accumulate and bacteria to grow. It is important to cough and deep breathe while at rest for long periods of time to keep our lungs healthy and ensure a good oxygen supply to the rest of our body. If a patient is debilitated we must do this for them by frequent turning. This also helps to prevent skin sores from the lack of oxygen at points where their bodies are causing the vessels to collapse and impede the blood flow.

Some definitions of interest:

• Asthma: a chronic disease, there is no cure for, where the airways contract, swell, and get clogged with mucous in response to an allergic reaction to pollen, etc., if it is the atopic type (usually beginning in childhood), or in response to all of these plus stress, exercise, cold air, or more, if it is the nonatopic type (beginning after the age of 35)

• Bronchitis: inflammation of the mucous membranes of the tracheobronchial tree

• Diaphragm: the layer of fibrous muscle that separates the thoracic cavity from the abdominal cavity

• Emphysema: a condition where the walls of the alveoli are overinflated and damaged causing a loss of lung elasticity and decreased gas exchange

• Hemoptysis: the coughing up of blood

• Pneumonia: inflammation of the lungs caused by bacteria, viruses, rickettsiae or fungi, or by inhalation of foreign material such as vomitus, where the alveoli become plugged with exudate (fluid or discharge)

• Sputum: a material coughed up from the lungs

• TB (tuberculosis): an infection, usually of the lungs, caused by an acid-fast bacillus that is inhaled or ingested, that causes severe illness and is highly contagious as long as it is present in the sputum

• Thorax: the cage of bones covering the lungs, heart, and part of the abdominal organs

THE DIGESTIVE SYSTEM

The gastrointestinal tract includes the whole digestive system, from the mouth to the anus. Digestion starts as soon as food or fluid enters the mouth through its breakdown by the saliva, and the absorption of some of its properties through the mucosa of the mouth. When food is chewed into small pieces and swallowed, it travels down the esophagus into the stomach where it is broken down further by hydrochloric acid. This liquefies food and slowly releases it into the small intestine. The **small intestine** is the longest part of the digestive tract, and is the major organ of absorption of prepared food. In addition to the mastication and hydrolysis, food is prepared for digestion by the intestinal secretions and enzymes that produce absorbable amino acids, emulsified fat particles, and monosaccharides.

Though the pancreas, liver, and gallbladder are not considered part of the gastrointestinal tract, I felt them important to include here, as they are involved in the process of digestion.

The **pancreas** is a gland, about 6 inches long, that sits longways between the kidneys in the epigastric area. It secretes digestive enzymes, insulin, and glucagon which aid in the breakdown of proteins into amino acids, breaks down fats, and converts starch into simple sugars.

The **liver** produces about a pint of bile daily, which is stored in the gallbladder, then released into the small intestine to break fats into small pieces to be digested. The liver also secretes glucose, proteins, vitamins, fats and others.

The **gallbladder** is a pear-shaped sac that sits on the surface of the right lobe of the liver. When it receives bile from the liver it concentrates and stores it. It contracts and releases bile into the small intestine during the digestion of fats. In this way, food is converted into absorbable nutrients that pass into intestinal cells. They are required in metabolism. A nutrient is a chemical substance that is essential for growth, reproduction, and maintenance of health. Metabolism is the chemical process in the distribution of nutrients in the blood after digestion.

The waste products continue on through the large intestine and out the anus by a rhythmic contraction of the smooth muscle of the intestine, called peristalsis. Dietary fiber is found in plant foods that are non-digestible carbohydrates. They effect the time it takes for wastes to move through the colon, water absorption, and the metabolism of fatty acids to serve as an energy reserve. (Regular consumption of fiber will help to decrease the risk of obesity, constipation, hemorrhoids, and colon cancer.)

Some definitions of interest:

• Alimentary tract: another name for the digestive tract

• Chyle: the cloudy liquid products of digestion transferred by the lymphatic system into the blood

• Digestion: the conversion of foods into absorbable substances

• Electrolyte: an element, found in different concentrations in plasma, interstitial fluid and cell fluid, that is able to conduct electric current (a proper balance of them is critical to normal metabolism)

• Emesis: vomit

• Feces: waste that is formed in the intestine and expelled through the rectum

• Gastric: pertaining to the stomach

• Heartburn: a burning sensation in the esophagus just below the area of the heart

• Hiatal hernia: where a portion of the stomach protrudes upward through the diaphragm causing the stomach contents to backflow into the esophagus

• Mastication: chewing food while it mixes with saliva

• Metabolize: to breakdown food stuffs into nutrients and eliminate the waste products

• Morbid Obesity: an excess of the body fat that threatens respiration and other body functions to the point that it threatens life

• Obese: body weight that is 20% over the desired weight for a person's age, height, sex and body build. The average human body is 25% fat. This is doubled for the medically defined obese person.

THE URINARY SYSTEM

The **kidneys** are two bean-shaped organs, sitting one on each side of the abdomen. Each one is about 5 inches long, 3 inches wide, and an inch or so thick. Their main structure for filtration and reabsorption is the **nephrons** (about 2 million of them). They filter the blood and eliminate wastes through the urine and return the purified plasma to the blood. Almost 1200 liters (quarts) of blood pass through the kidneys every day. All the blood in the body passes through the kidneys about 20 times per hour, though only about 1/5 of it is filtered through the nephrons. With the help of hormones, they work to maintain the fluid and electrolyte balance. The **antidiuretic** hormone is produced by the pituitary gland and is the major hormone involved with regulating the water-electrolyte balance of the body. Each kidney has a tube about 15 inches long, called a ureter, that carries urine from the kidney to the bladder. A small tubular structure, called a urethra, drains urine from the bladder out of the body.

Some definitions of interest:

• Anuria: cessation of urine production (less than 100 ml/day

• Ascites: an accumulation of fluid in the peritoneal cavity

• Cystitis: inflammation of the bladder and ureters

• Dialysis: diffusion of particles from areas of high to lower concentration to remove unwanted substances from the blood

• Edema: accumulation of fluid in interstitial spaces of tissues (between the tissue cells)

• Electrolyte: an element or compound that separates into ions and is able to conduct an electric current (sodium, potassium, chloride, magnesium)

• Enuresis: incontinence of urine

• Foley: a catheter that is placed in the bladder to drain the urine into a collection bag

• Nephritis: inflammation of the kidneys

• Oliguria: diminished urine output (less than 500 ml/day

• Renal: pertaining to the kidneys

• Renal failure: when the kidneys fail to concentrate the urine, conserve electrolytes, and excrete wastes as they should

• Uremia: excessive amounts of nitrogenous waste, such as urea, in the blood. This occurs in renal failure. Measured by the BUN (blood urea nitrogen)

• UTI (Urinary tract infection): an infection of one or more of the structures of the urinary system

THE REPRODUCTIVE SYSTEM

The reproductive system includes all of the male and female external genitalia, ducts and glands that function to create offsring. For this system I have chosen to merely define the separate parts, as I have found that to even begin to detail the sequence of this system is a book in and of itself!

Female:

• Clitoris: vaginal erectile structure found outside of and above the vaginal canal

• Fallopian tubes: a pair of ducts that open into the uterus at one end, and over the ovaries at the other, that serve as a passage where an ovum is carried to the uterus

• Ovaries: a pair of female gonads, one on each side of the uterus, that secrete hormones to regulate the menstrual cycle, and release eggs (ovum) for fertilization by sperm

• Uterus: the pear-shaped, hollow, female organ where the fertilized egg is implanted and fetus is developed

• Vagina: the canal from the orifice (opening) of the female genitalia to the cervix of the uterus

• Vulva: the skin of the labia, clitoris, and surrounding tissues

Male:

• Ejaculatory duct: the duct that goes from the seminal vesicles to the ductus deferens through which semen enters the urethra

• Epididymis: one of a pair of ducts that carry sperm from the testes to the vas deferens

• Penis: the male external erectile reproductive organ

• Prostate: a male gland that produces a secretion that liquefies coagulated semen. It is about the size of a chestnut and sits at the base of the penis, and surrounds the neck of the bladder and base of the urethra

• Seminal vesicles: a pair of glandular structures, sitting behind the male bladder, that produce a fluid that is added to other secretions to form the semen (sperm)

• Testes: a pair of gonads, suspended in the scrotum, that produce sperm and testosterone

• Vas deferens: the tube-like structures that extend from the epididymis and join the seminal vesicles to form the ejaculatory duct

Some more definitions of interest:

• Estrogen: a hormone that promotes the female secondary sex characteristics

• Gonads: reproductive glands (ovaries and testes)

• Hysterectomy: removal of the uterus

• Menopause: when the menses (menstrual period) stops; frequently referred to as the period when the hormone levels change causing hot flashes and mood swings

• Oophorectomy: removal of the ovaries

• Spontaneous abortion: miscarriage

• Testosterone: a hormone that promotes the male secondary sex characteristics

• TURP (transurethral resection of the prostate): removal of the prostate through the urethra

• Vasectomy: cutting or removal of the vas deferens to cause infertility

THE ENDOCRINE SYSTEM

This system is made-up of several ductless glands that produce and secrete hormones directly into the bloodstream or lymph nodes and effect the function of their target organs. These glands are the pineal gland, hypothalamus, the anterior and posterior pituitary, thyroid and parathyroid, the pancreas, the adrenal glands and the gonads.

The **pineal gland** is located in the brain. It secretes the hormone, called melatonin, that causes drowsiness. It secretes as much as 10 times more at night than during the day. It also decreases skin pigmentation (skin color), and inhibits (blocks) the effects of some other endocrine functions, such as the gonad hormones. Some people take an over-the-counter preparation of melatonin to help them sleep, and some believe it to have antiaging effects.

The **hypothalamus** is located in the brain. It controls the peripheral autonomic nervous system (see the section on nerves), endocrine processes, and many of the somatic (body) functions such as temperature, sleep, and appetite.

The **pituitary glands** are located at the base of the brain. They produce the somatotropin (growth) hormone, prolactin (aids in the growth and development of the mammary glands), thyroid stimulating hormone, follicle stimulating hormone (growth and maturation of the ovaries and sperm), luteinizing hormone (maturation and secretion of sex hormones), adrenocorticotropic hormone (stimulates the secretion of steroids), melanocyte stimulating hormone (controls the amount of melanin produced), vasopressin (antidiuretic hormone, decreases the production of urine) and oxytocin (stimulates the contraction of the uterus).

The **thyroid gland** is located at the front of the neck, folded over the trachea, forming two lobes. It produces thyroxin and calcitonin. These hormones increase the rate of metabolism, maintain the secretion of the growth hormone, maintain the heart's rate and force, aid in skeletal maturation, promote the development of the central nervous system, are necessary for muscle tone, and affect the body temperature.

The **parathyroids** are a group of several small glands, attached to the thyroid gland, that secrete the parathyroid hormone. It helps to maintain the concentration of calcium in the blood. It is essential for normal neuromuscular irritability and blood clotting.

The **pancreas** secretes insulin (for the metabolism of glucose, fats, carbohydrates and proteins), glucagon (for the conversion of glycogen to glucose), and pancreatic polypeptide (for growth, development and maintenance of health), and several other hormones associated with the regulation of cellular metabolism.

The **adrenal glands**, also known as the suprarenal glands, sit on top of each kidney. They secrete androgens (for the development of testosterone and estrogen), cortisol (for inflammation), aldosterone (to retain sodium, conserve water, and excrete potassium), epinephrine (a vasoconstrictor), and norepinephrine (to constrict the vessels and increase the blood pressure).

The **gonads** are the reproductive glands; ovaries and testes (see the reproductive system).

Some definitions of interest:

• Diabetes insipidus: a metabolic disorder where there is not enough of the anti-diuretic hormone, causing too much urine to be excreted, or the kidneys are unable to respond to the anti-diuretic hormones

• Diabetes Mellitus: a disease caused by the body producing little or no insulin, or the inability of the body to use the insulin, causing glucose (blood sugar) to collect in the blood. Insulin-dependent (type 1) occurs when the pancreas makes too little or none. Non-insulin dependent (type 2) occurs when insulin is made, but the body is unable to use it effectively

• Dialysis: separation of impurities from the body by diffusion through a membrane

• Fistula: passage of an organ to the surface, or between two organs. One is surgically made by connecting an artery to a vein for the purpose of hemodialysis

• Grave's disease: a disorder where the thyroid gland is usually enlarged and too much hormones is produced, causing nervousness, weight loss, fatigue, and an increased metabolic rate and heat intolerance

• Hypothyroidism: decreased activity of the thyroid gland. May cause mental and physical lethargy, weight gain, constipation, dry skin, and arthritis

• Myxedema: a condition caused by untreated hypothyroidism that leads to coma and death

• Pancreatitis: inflammation of the pancreas causing abdominal and back pain, fever, nausea and vomiting, and a loss of appetite

• Thyroid storm: where the thyroid releases too much hormones and causes a crisis of a very high fever, fast heart rate, extreme shortness of breath, anxiety, and could even cause coma or death

MEDICATION INFORMATION

Many of the same drugs are made by different companies. The GENERIC name is the one given to that particular drug or compound, and the BRAND name is the one given to it by the company that makes it. Drugs are regulated by the FDA and have to be made of the same substance and quality in order to pass their strict standards. Therefore, when you buy a brand name drug you will more than likely pay more for it than if you bought the generic. For example: the generic name for aspirin is acetylsalicylic acid. Some of the brand names are Bayer and Ecotrin. You can sometimes get 2-10 times the amount of the same drug for the same price if you buy the generic.

Most drugs are metabolized in the liver and excreted by the kidneys. Therefore, their effects differ in the very young due to underdeveloped metabolic and renal function, and the very old due to their diminished metabolic and renal function. Also, there are many diseases that effect the absorption, metabolism, and excretion of drugs. Always let your doctor know all of the drugs that you are, or plan to be, taking. You should know the names of your drugs, why you are taking them, the time of day you are to take your medicine for proper therapeutic use, as well as how to store it (in tight containers, away from sunlight and extreme temperatures).

As you know, your pharmacist gives you printed information on your medicines when you pick them up. This information also includes drugs and foods that should not be taken together and/or the effects they will have if you do.

You may not know that a lot of them have a computer program that will list the drugs and foods that you should not take together, the things you should watch out for (side effects), and the things you should do or not do based on your age, height, weight and any health problems you have, making it tailored to you. Ask them if they have this program, then give them all of the information you can. This is important information and must be followed in order to get the effect you desire.

An adverse reaction of a drug is an effect other than what is therapeutically intended. If it is mild and predictable it is called an **adverse effec**t. If the adverse reaction is hazardous the doctor may discontinue the drug or lower its dose. A drug **allergy** is one that you are hypersensitive to and is the result of an immune reaction. Some of these are fatal (it can kill you). **An upset stomach is not an allergic reaction, swelling in the throat is!**

Drug toxicities are those caused by a level of that drug in your blood that your body can not handle. Most of them are dose related and readily reversible with adjustment of the dose. These are some of the things that will be listed on your pharmacy printout as things to watch out for. Make sure that you tell your nurse and/or doctor of any undesired reaction you may have to any drug.

Some drugs must be adjusted according to blood levels in order to maintain the desired effect, and to prevent an undesired one. A good example of this is with Coumadin. It prevents the action of the clotting factors formed in the liver. People who are on Coumadin are potential "free bleeders" because their blood does not form clots as usual. They must have their blood drawn at least once a month to check their prothrombin (PT) level. In your maintenance log I have included a sheet for you to write down your doctor or lab appointments. I also included a space for you to log the results if you are lucky, or persistent, enough to know them. Log such things as your PT/PTT if you are on coumadin; your Hct/Hgb if you are anemic; T-Cell count if you have HIV; etc.

FREQUENTLY USED TERMS

B.I.D. = Twice a day

H.S. = At bedtime

I.M. = Intramuscular

I.V. = Intravenous

P.O. = By mouth

P.R.N. = As needed (no set time)

Q DAY= Every day

Q.I.D. = Four times/day

T.I.D. = Three times/day

TABLE OF EQUIVALENTS

1 teaspoon (tsp) = 5 ml or cc

1 tablespoon (T or Tbs) = 15 ml or cc

1 fluid ounce = 30 ml or cc

1 cup = 240 ml or cc

1 pint = 473 ml or cc

1 quart = 946 ml or cc

1 liter = 1000 ml or cc

1 milliliter (ml) = 1000 microliters (ul)

1 cubic centimer (cc) = 1 milliliter (ml)

1 kilogram (kg) = 1000 grams (G or gm)

1 gram (G) = 1000 mlligrams (mg

1 milligram (mg) = 1000 micrograms (mcg)

1 ounce (oz) = 30 grams (G)

1 pound (lb) = 453.6 grams (G)

1 kilogram (kg) = 2.2 pounds (lbs)

1 centimeter = 0.3937 inch (in)

IMPROVE YOUR ODDS

We all gamble with our lives from the moment we get up in the morning. But some of these we do to ourselves... on purpose. If you want to improve your odds, start with the reason that most people are admitted to the hospital... Heart disease **Heart disease** is the most common risk factor for all of us. The most common risks are family **history, age, obesity, lack of physical activity, high cholesterol, high blood pressure, diabetes** and, of course, **smoking**. You can't do anything about your **family history**, but you can do something about your future family's history. If you are at a higher risk because your father or brother had heart disease before they were 55, or your mother or sister before 65, keep your cholesterol, blood pressure, and diabetes under control to help improve the odds for your children!!

As much as we would all like, we can't do anything about our **age**. Except thrive to gain more of it! We have become a nation of obese men, women and children! What are we doing to our children? How many times have you looked at a 10-year-old and thought, "that kid's parents should be ashamed. Don't they know he'll probably die before he reaches adulthood?" His poor little heart is having to work overtime just to haul it around. Consumption of more food than the body needs, and the wrong kinds of foods, results in an increase in fat storage and the build-up of fatty deposits in our blood, causing narrowing or clogging of the arteries.

Heart failure does not happen over night, as the weakened heart strains harder and harder, over time it stretches the heart fibers and causes the heart to be larger and weaker. Chronic heart failure takes a long time to develop, and though the symptoms can be controlled with diligence, it can not be cured.

Lack of physical activity is one of the reasons people become obese. A good exercise program can reduce your risk of heart disease and stroke, improve your body's ability to use oxygen, and improve the blood circulation. It also helps lower the "bad" cholesterol and increase the "good" cholesterol, and it helps you sleep better and handle more stress. Walking may sound simple, but it is a great way to get the exercise you need. It keeps the body toned and the circulation healthy. It's not necessary to jog or lift weights, but do something besides sitting or lying. If you feel you need or want more exercise, and you have a medical condition that limits your activities in any way, ask your doctor about your limits.

High cholesterol is more of a common risk factor these days. We're in a hurry, so fast food has become very popular. One of the fastest ways to prepare food is to fry it - in fat! Of course, there are other foods high in cholesterol, like my favorites mayonnaise and butter. Your total cholesterol level should be below 200mg/dl (milligrams per deciliter of blood). We know that there is "good" and "bad" cholesterol. The low-density lipoprotein, LDL, increases the risk of build-up in the arteries.

The high-density lipoprotein, HDL, reduces the build-up in the arteries by removing the extra cholesterol in the blood. The LDL should be less than 160, preferably below 100. An HDL of 60 or above will help protect against heart disease.

Triglycerides are very low density lipoproteins. Though they are a major energy source, they are the most common type of fat in your blood, and high levels will increase your risk of heart disease. Your level should be less than 150mg/dl. Control your weight, exercise regularly, and eat a well balanced diet of foods low in saturated fat and cholesterol such as fish, lean meats, fruits and vegetables, whole grains and potatoes, fat-free milk and cheese, angel food cake and fig bars.

In your maintenance log, you will find a sheet for "frequent measurements" and one for "doctor or laboratory appointments". Choose one of these forms and keep track of your cholesterol. Your doctor may also have you on a medication to help lower your cholesterol, such as Lipitor or Zocor. These are not miracle drugs, they must be taken over a period of time, and you must still diet and exercise if you want to see an improvement.

High blood pressure is caused by pressure in the arteries being too high. This causes them to not stretch easily and the left ventricle in the heart has to strain harder to pump the blood out. Over a period of time, the heart becomes enlarged and weak, resulting in heart failure. ACE(angiotensin-converting enzyme) inhibitors are drugs that limit the amount of angiotensin in our bodies.

Angiotensin is a substance made in our bodies that tighten our arteries. Therefore, the ACE inhibitors (like Capoten, Vasotec, Accupril, Altace, and Lisinopril) help relax them, lowering blood pressure. If your doctor determines that you should not take an ACE inhibitor, he may prescribe an angiotensin II blocker (Losartan or Valsartan) or a vasodilator (Isordil or Hydralasine).

If you've had high blood pressure for a while, and the doctor determines that you have some heart failure, he may add a betablocker. Remember the endocrine system? The adrenal glands secrete norepinephrine to constrict the vessels and increase the blood pressure. Well, beta-blockers (Coreg or Toprol) block the effect of the norepinephrine. This releases the pressure on the arteries, lowering the blood pressure, decreasing demand on the heart. The heart rate then slows down and pumps more effectively. It may take months for these drugs to have the desired effect, and they should never be stopped without a doctor's advice. Diuretics (Lasix or Bumex) are given to get rid of excess fluid by making the kidneys make more urine, and this will also lower blood pressure. Most diuretics cause you to lose potassium through the urine, so you may require a potassium supplement to ensure that the heart rhythm is controlled.

Diabetes is the common name for Diabetes Mellitus. It is a disease caused by the body producing too little or no insulin, or the inability of the body to use the insulin, causing glucose to collect in the blood. Because this is such a common disease, and becoming more common every day, diabetic education has become a priority in the medical field. For this reason, and the fact that it would make a book in itself, I will say no more than keep it under control. If you are diabetic, you know the things you should do to control it. You must follow the diet and medication regimen your doctor has set. It does not work to take extra insulin because you chose to eat extra sugars! You are killing yourself. It's not your fault that you have it, and we all know it can't be cured, but it can be controlled. If you do not keep your diabetes under control you WILL develop other body system diseases.

The Surgeon General warns us against **smoking.** Many believe the smoke that is breathed-in by by-standers is as dangerous to them as the inhaled smoke is to the smoker. For this reason, it has become against the law to smoke in some (most) public areas. It has become a topic of much debate across the USA, especially in the workplace. Smoking is very addictive. Those of us who have been unfortunate enough to have the habit know just how hard it is to quit, even with the facts staring us in the eye. The choice to quit must be just that; a choice. We also need the support of those who care, just as people who are addicted to any other drug do. Yes, tobacco is a drug. In fact it is many of them all rolled-up (forgive the pun) in one.

I'll list them here, and you decide how important it is **To-Smoke-Or-Not-To-Smoke**!

Acetone: a volatile solvent (found in nail polish remover).

Ammonia: makes people more suseptable to viral illness.

Benzene: a solvent in fuel. It causes cancer, especially leukemia.

Cadmium: a poisonous metal (used to make batteries). It causes liver, kidney, and brain damage.

Carbon Monoxide: a poisonous gas that causes an increase in the heart rate and shortness of breath. It attaches itself to the red blood cells so they can't carry oxygen.

Formaldehyde: a poisonous liquid (used to preserve dead bodies) It causes respiratory, skin, and gastrointestional problems, as well as cancer.

Hydrogen Cyanide: a toxic gas that causes headaches, dizziness, nausea, and vomiting.

Lead: a toxic heavy metal that causes damage to the brain, kidneys, nervous system, and red blood cells. It also causes birth defects and learning disabilities.

Nicotine: causes cigarettes to be as addictive as cocaine and heroine.

Tar: paralyses the small hairs (cilia) that protect and clean the lungs.

THIS EASY

You give me love
You've lifted me up
You fill me

You light up my life
Made me your wife
You thrill me

Always been there
To show me you care
You love me

One of a kind
You're a valuable find
You touch me

I promise to try
To be the best wife
I can be

I'll do my part
To earn your heart
You will see

'Til the day I die
Not a day will go by
Believe me

That I won't pray
We will always stay
This easy

Constance Hope Stringer
To my husband, Glenn
1998

Chapter Seven
CAUSES OF DEATH

According to the National Center for Health Statistics' (NCSH) 2002 report, the 10 leading causes of death for all ages in 2002 were heart disease, followed by cancer, then strokes, chronic lower respiratory diseases, accidents, diabetes, pneumonia and flu, alzheimers, kidney disease, then septicemia. Below I have outlined these and others of interest. I have included some of the statistics from the NCSH 2002 report. Keep in mind that these figures can change from year to year, mainly because of the AIDS epidemic.

HEART DISEASE is defined by Webster as: "any pathological or abnormal condition of the heart". It is the leading cause of death in those 65 and older; Second for those 45-64. Below are some of the related conditions. I have put them in alphabetical order; not necessarily in order of severity or danger.

Aneurysm: the widening of a blood vessel in an area that has become stretched or weakened, causing a sac that is filled with blood. The blood may clot and become an embolism or the vessel may rupture causing uncontrolled bleeding. The extent of the danger is measured by the size and location of the aneurysm.

Aortic Valve Disorder: The aorta is the main artery coming from the left ventricle of the heart. Its' valve is a fold of membranous tissue that prevents the blood from flowing backward into the ventricle. When the valve is too loose or too hard it can not preform its' duties and the heart becomes congested and the body does not get the blood flow it needs.

Aortic Stenosis: Scar tissue, caused from infection or rheumatic fever, causes the aorta to become narrowed and the pressure in the aorta becomes too high to handle the amount of blood pumped into it from the heart.

Cardic death: When the heart stops beating.

Cardiac dysrhythmia: An abnormal rhythm of the heart beat. Ventricular tachycardia is a lethal rhythm where the heart beats too fast to sustain life and it is often followed by sudden cardiac death.

Coronary Atherosclerosis: When lipid deposits accumulate within one of the coronary vessels. Large accumulations may cause the arteries to become occluded.

Endocarditis: Inflammation of the inner lining of the heart muscle in reaction to injury or irritation. This may cause loss of function of the heart.

Heart Block: An altered heart rhythm caused by an impairment of the normal electrical conduction pathways in the heart. There are different degrees of heart block, the most dangerous of which is complete heart block.

Heart Failure: When the heart is not able to maintain sufficient circulation to the body resulting in the heart stopping. Left heart failure is where the left ventricle is not pumping effectively and blood backs up into the lungs. Right heart failure is where the right ventricle is not pumping effectively and blood and fluid back up into the general circulation.

Myocardial Infarction: (heart attack) Damage to part of the heart muscle caused by obstruction of the blood flow in an artery that supplies that part of the heart. This often causes sudden cardiac death.

CANCER is defined by Webster as: "a malignant tumor; neoplasm; sarcoma or carcinoma characterized by abnormal growth of cells which spread to other tissues". It is the leading cause of death in those 45 to 64; Second in those 5-14 and 35-45. Below I have listed some of the types of cancer in alphabetical order; not necessarily in the order of severity or danger. Keep in mind that benign tumors are are relatively undangerous, where malignant tumors are those that resist treatment and threaten to cause death. Benign tumors often end with the suffix "oma" where the malignant ones end with "sarcoma" or "carcinoma". For our purposes here I will only list those that are malignant.

Adenocarcinoma: malignant cancer of the glandular epithelium (the coverings of specified glands).

Angiosarcoma: malignant cancer of blood vessels.

Basal Cell Carcinoma: a malignant type of skin cancer.

Chondrosarcoma: malignant cancer of the cartilage.

Cholangiocarcinoma: malignant cancer of the bile duct.

Glioblastoma: malignant cancer of the nerve tissue.

Hepatocellular Carcinoma: malignant cancer of the liver.

Hemangiosarcoma: malignant cancer of blood vessels.

Hodgkin's Disease: malignant cancer of the lymphoid tissues.

Leiomyosarcoma: malignant cancer of smooth muscles.

Leukemia: malignant cancer of the leucocytes in the blood forming organs of the body.

Liposarcoma: malignant cancer of fat.

Lymphangiosarcoma: malignant cancer of the lymph vessels.

Malignant Meningioma: malignant cancer of the membranes enveloping the spinal cord and brain.

Medulloblastoma: malignant cancer of the medulla of the brain.

Multiple Myeloma: malignant cancer originating in the cells of the bone marrow.

Neuroblastoma: malignant cancer of the nerve cells.

Osteogenic Sarcoma: malignant cancer of the bone.

Renal Cell Carcinoma: malignant cancer of the kidney.

Rhabdomyosarcoma: malignant cancer of striated muscle.

Seminoma: malignant cancer of the testis.

Some cancers are named after that part of the body it inhabits, such as lung cancer and breast cancer.

STROKES are cerebrovascular accidents caused by a lack of oxygenated blood to a part of the brain brought on by occlusion or rupture of a vessel in that part of the brain. It is the third leading cause of death in those 65 and older. The symptoms vary greatly depending on the location of the injury to the brain, and the severity of that injury. The symptoms may resolve themselves in a matter of minutes, or they may last a lifetime. If the injury is severe enough it can cause sudden death, or the person may be left without any number of senses such as speech, sight, or movement of limbs. In most cases some of the memory is lost. If the stroke is due to a blood clot, and treatment is sought within the first two to three hours, the clot can be disolved with thrombolytics.

Medications like Heparin and Coumadin can prevent clots from forming, but once formed it requires medications that are very expensive and risky in order to disolve them.

People with high blood pressure are especially at risk for strokes and heart attacks. Plaque, a build-up of cholesterol and other materials, narrows the arteries and can restrict the flow of blood. High blood pressure puts stress on these areas and may cause it to rupture.

When there is a break in a vessel platelets stick together to form a clot in order to seal the "leak". A thrombus is a stationary clot.

An embolus is a clot or other material that has broken off and travels to other areas. When this embolus becomes lodged in a vessel in the heart and occludes the blood flow there it causes a heart attack. When this embolus becomes lodged in a vessel in the brain it causes a stroke, also known as a cerebrovascular accident.

Some early signs of a stroke are 1) sudden numbness or weakness in the face, an arm, or a leg. 2) sudden confusion 3) sudden trouble speaking or understanding 4) sudden blurry, or loss of, vision 5) sudden loss of balance 6) sudden difficulty swallowing. If any of these symptoms develop you should seek immediate medical assistance.

LOWER RESPIRATORY DISEASES are a group of diseases effecting the lungs. This group of diseases is known as chronic obstructive pulmonary disease (COPD) or chronic lower respiratory disease (CLRD). It is the third leading cause of death in those 55 to 64. A leading cause of preventable disease and death in the United States is cigarette smoking.

ACCIDENTS are the 5th overall leading cause of death in our country; the leading cause in those 1-44; and third in those 45-54. This group includes motor vehicle accidents, poisonings, falls, suffocations, drownings, fires, natural disasters, and firearms. How careless!

DIABETES is the sixth leading cause of overall deaths; fourth in those 55-64. It is a disease caused by the pancreas either not making enough insulin, or not being able to use the insulin to help get the sugar from food into the body cells. When this happens the sugar stays in the blood causing the person to be very thirsty, urinate often, feel hungry and tired, have dry skin, have slow healing sores, have numbness in the feet, and have blurry eyesight. Left untreated, diabetes can cause serious problems with your eyes, kidneys, nerves, and blood vessels.

Most people should have a blood sugar of 70-150. Though it goes up after a meal, it should return to normal after 1-2 hours. If you have diabetes your doctor will tell you what range he wants your blood sugar to remain in, how often to check your levels, and how to treat it. Some people can control their diabetes with diet and exercise, while others must take a pill or shot.

People with diabetes are more likely to develop high blood pressure, high cholesterol and fat levels, and heart disease. It is also the main cause of blindness in adults in the US. The high blood sugar level causes bleeding in the blood vessels of the eye. Diabetes is also the main cause of kidney failure. Nerve damage in the feet caused by diabetes is a main cause of amputations.

High blood sugar leads to infections, and infections cause the blood sugar to rise even higher! You can see how this can effect the whole body. It is very important that diabetes be kept under control. In order to do this you must do all of these things every day: eat healthy food, get regular exercise, test your blood sugar, and take your diabetes medicine.

PNEUMONIA AND FLU are especially dangerous for the elderly and very young. They are the seventh leading overall cause of death; fifth in those 65 and over; and sixth in those 1-4. These infections of the resiratory tract are hard on the body, and if the person is not able to fight off that infection it could lead to death. Of course, not as many people actually die from them as they use to, with our current technology, but the numbers remain high. The flu and pneumonia vaccines should be taken regularly by the very young and the very old.

ALZHEIMER'S is a form of dementia that is often mistaken for normal signs of aging. It ranks eighth overall, and sixth in those 65 and over. It is a debilitating disease that is often terminal. We are still not sure of the cause, and there is currently no cure, but there are some medications that help improve the symptoms. Below is a general summary of the progression of alzheimers'. You can see how early treatment is necessary:

Symptoms are mild for the first 2-4 years. Memory loss is evident; they repeat themselves; they get lost and lose things; and personality changes begin. Some support is needed.

Symptoms are moderate the next 2-10 years. They lose their recent memory; have difficulty dressing themselves and doing simple tasks; forget to shower; argue alot; wander; worry and are depressed alot; beleive things are real that aren't. Close supervision is required.

Symptoms are severe the next 1-3 years. They can't use or understand words; don't recognize themselves or family members; can't care for themselves; can't control their bowel or bladder. Total care is required.

KIDNEY DISEASE can cause high blood pressure, anemia, high cholesterol, depression and sexual dysfunction. It ranks nineth overall and eighth in those 65 and older. The kidneys remove waste products and excess fluids from the body, as well as maintain a balance of salt, potassium and acid. They also produce a hormone that stimulates the production of red blood cells, and other hormones that help regulate calcium metabolism and blood pressure.

Because each of the kidney's functions can be effected seperately, urine output can be normal even with severe kidney disease. Early diagnosis and treatment of kidney problems can prevent multiple body system diseases. These days a great number of people live reasonably normal lives, and much longer, with dialysis and kidney transplants.

SEPTICEMIA is blood poisoning, usually with a bacteria. Though tenth overall, it is the seventh leading cause of death in those 65 and older. It is a medical emergency that requires immediate medical treatment. Around 20% of those with septicemia die. Those effected often have tiny blood spots on the skin that look like pin pricks. This is called a hemorrhagic rash. Left untreated, they begin to get bigger until they look like fresh bruises that eventually join together to form large areas of discoloration. Septicemia develops rapidly and the patient becomes very ill with a fever, lose interest in things, develop cold feet and hands, and may go into a coma and die. Swift treatment with antibiotic therapy is necessary. It is the 10th leading cause of death in the USA.

LIVER DISEASE is the fourth leading cause of death in those 45-54; seventh in those 35-44; and tenth in those 25-34. The build-up of fat in the liver cells can cause inflammation of the liver, which can lead to scarring and hardening of the liver. Fatty Liver is caused by obesity, vitamin A toxicity, drugs, alcohol, diabetes mellitus, and high triglycerides. Long term use of toxic substances, such as alcohol, can cause further injury and a condition known as Cirrhosis.

The scarring, also called fibrosis, blocks the bile ducts causing the bile to back-up into the liver and bloodstream. It may also block the blood flow to the liver causing a condition called portal hypertension.

SUICIDE is the second leading cause of death in those 25-34; third in those 10-24; fourth in those 35-44; fifth in those 45-54; and eighth in those 55-64. You can see by these numbers that a great number of people in our society are affected with hopelessness, depression, and substance abuse. We all need to work a little harder to ensure that our fellow human-beings' needs are met.

HOMICIDE is the second leading cause of death in those 15-24; third in those 1-4 and 25-34; fourth in those 5-9; fifth in those 10-14; and sixth in those 35-44. This is the intentional death of another for ones' own gain. What will become of a society that takes the lives of so many others. This is no way to be fruitfull and multiply.

HIV was the fifth leading cause of death in those 35-44 in 2002; sixth in those 25-34; and eighth in those 15-24 and 45-54. AIDS stands for Acquired Immune Deficiency Syndrome. It is caused by the Human Immunodeficiency Virus. If you get infected with the virus your body will make antibodies to fight it. It is this antibody that is detected when you are tested for HIV, but it can take 3-6 months to detect the antibody after you have become infected with HIV. During this time you can be infecting others and not even know it.

You can get HIV from anyone who is infected by having sex with them; sharing a needle with them; having their blood come in contact with any open wound (even a scratch) you may have; being born by an infected mother, or drinking her breast milk. The risk of receiving an infected persons' blood through transfusion is very low these days because of our strict screening of the blood supply.

You are not considered to have AIDS until your immune system is damaged to the point that your CD4+ cells (T-helper cells) fall below 200 or below 14% .The virus multiplies quickly and, as it wears down your immune system, it makes it harder to fight off any other virus, bacteria, fungus or parasite you may come in contact with. Any one of these antigens could cause what is called an "opportunistic infection". The CDC lists the most common ones as: a lung infection called Pneumocystis Pneumonia (PCP); a skin cancer called Kaposi's Sarcoma (KS); an infection of the eyes called Cytomegalovirus (CMV); and a fungal infection of the throat or vagina called Candida. People usually die of AIDS-related infections.

Because not all places are required to report an HIV diagnosis; many people are not aware that they are infected; and many of those who do know found out by using a home test kit, there is no way to know just how many people are infected. A great number of people die of an AIDS-related illness without ever being tested for AIDS.

LIKE THE SUN

Though in my actions it may not show
And my words can't tell its worth
My love for you continues to grow
Reaching heights of none on Earth

You're in my thoughts day and night
If only I could tell you so
But I can't find the words that are right
I can only hope, dear, that you know

You know I love you and always will
But I wish I could make you see
Just how deeply this love I feel
How very much you mean to me

It warms my heart when you are near
Oh, the joy that loving you holds
But knowing that you also hold me dear
Like the sun, warms my very soul

Constance Hope Stringer
To my husband, Glenn
2005

Chapter Eight
THE HARD PART

Euphemisms, such as he "expired", he "passed on", or he "is gone", tend to confuse people and leave room for doubt. Death is final. It is a fact that must be faced. In our attempts to be kind and comforting it is the manner in which we state the facts, not the avoidance of them, that is most effective. We must educate ourselves as best we can in order to lower our anxieties about death so that we can better treat the emotional issues of the dying patient in our care, not just the physical. It is the spiritual issues that most people have a hard time with. Most of us have used the expression, "He has gone to a better place". But how many of us have said it with conviction? What do you really believe about "life after death"? Sure, no one really knows any particulars about heaven. How could we? Are the streets paved with gold? Are the gates really of pearl? Will we be able to touch the hand of God? The good thing is that none of those things matter. What really matters is that we believe in God, what ever language we use to identify him.

I am a Christian. I do not preach it. Maybe I should. Haven't we been taught to "spread the word"? I'm not ashamed of it, by any means. If the subject comes up I'm one of the first to join the conversation, but I don't initiate it without prompting. There are those who have been called to preach (and those who do harm to the institution of religion by exploiting it for their own means).

There are those who try to shove it down our throats, and only leave a bad taste in the mouths of those who resent it. I think that religion and spirituality is something that people must decide for themselves, then ponder on awhile. Self reflection is the only way we will learn about our own beliefs and values. I have had God in my heart for as long as I can remember. I remember being a very young girl and having long conversations with God. I use to talk to him about the simplest things, as if he were in the room with me. I regret to say that I don't do that as often as I use to, but I still know that, when I do, he listens. I know beyond a shadow of a doubt that there is a heaven. Call it blind faith, if you will. But I don't need any more proof of God's existance than that I feel him. I like the way that feels. If the rest of the world felt this feeling they'd be hooked, too.

Look where the world is heading. Look where it has gone in the past 20 years; 10; 5. Can you honestly say that if everyone did unto others as they would like to have done unto them that it wouldn't be "heaven-here-on-earth"? No one wants to be killed, robbed, raped, hit, lied to, and lied about!

God has many names, in many different cultures. The important thing is that we all know that God, in any language, is **GOOD**, and that the devil, in any language is **BAD**.

I would hope that you have lead a good life, but it is never too late to start. Even on your deathbed. Think about the bad things you have done in your life, no matter how small. If it hurt anyone in any way, are you sorry for that pain? There are people that are inherently evil. That will do harm to any one, in any way, if it benefits them in any way, and they are not sorry! God wouldn't want them in his heaven, anymore than we want them on our earth. We, and He, must protect the innocent. Are you inherently evil? No? Then you may go to God's heaven just for the asking!

I have gone into this subject, not to shove-it-down-your-throat, but because it is an issue that may come up if the dying person has a good rapport with you. It is important that you know where you stand. If you do not believe in God, please step aside at this time. If he does not believe, or at least want to believe, he will not bring the subject up. If he does, then he will need your support, your conviction. Please do not tell a dying person that they believe in fairtales, and that none of them

71

have a happy ending. Because the happy ending to every life is but a new beginning!

Ok, I've brought up God in different cultures. Did you really believe that only caucasions, born and raised here in America, are God's children? God made everyone! And even those of us in the same cities have different religions, let alone those in other countries. And, face it, America is, more than ever, the "melting-pot". You may be the caregiver of someone who has a religion or culture other than yours. This is not the time to convert them. That they believe in God is enough. But it would be nice if you knew something about their religion, their culture. So I will outline some of them here (in alphabetical order), and hope that you care enough to find out more. Maybe the dying person would like to be the one to educate you; and be touched by the fact that you care that much.

Buddhists consider death an "awakening" where the dead is reborn. After death, other Buddhists do a good deed to show his thanks. They may even donate some of the deceased's belongings to ensure a good rebirth and enlightenment.

Catholicism is the largest christian religion in the world. It has been practiced since the time of Apostle Peter, who lived in the time of Jesus. The Pope in Rome administers the church's affairs through Priests and Bishops.

The Catholic's regular worship service is called the Mass. They observe the seven sacraments of: Eucharist (the communion); Baptism (the cleansing of the soul); Confirmation (the reaffirmation of the faith); Penance (the confession); Holy Orders (the ordination into priesthood); Matrimony (marriage sanctioned by the church); and Extreme Unction (annointing of the dying). Catholics are given "last rights" by a priest before they die. After death, the funeral is incorporated into the Mass.

Hinduism has been practiced in India since 1500 years before Christ. It includes many sects of the Indian people. Many of them believe in the "caste system"; they believe they are born into a subgroup that determines their religion, social standing and work duties (Priests, rulers, warriors, farmers, merchants, peasants or laborers). Hindus worship deities at shrines, and believe that the Divine Trinity is: Brahma the creator; Shiva the destoyer; and Vishnu the preserver. The Hindus believe in rebirth after death, but they believe they are released from repeated reincarnation through yoga and devotion to their guru. When a Hindu dies their bodies will be washed, wrapped in a shroud, surrounded with flowers, and family members will carry it to the funeral pyre for cremation.

Islam was founded by the Prophet Mohammed 600 years after Christ. Islam is Arabic for "submission to God", and the word for God is "Allah". The followers of Islam are Muslim. There are two main divisions of Islam; the Sunni (pronounced: soony) and the Shiite (pronounced: she-eye-t). It is common for Muslims to cremate their dead.

Jehovah's Witnesses believe that all members are ministers. They go door-to-door preaching their faith. They refuse to be members of the armed forces, refuse to salute national flags, and will not participate in politics. They believe that the second coming of Christ is imminent.

Judaism, founded 2000 years before Christ, is based on the Old Testament, which is the Hebrew bible (especially the part known as the Torah). The Orthodox Jews believe that the Torah is absolutely binding; the Reformed Jews believe in the ethical content of the Torah; the Conservative Jews allow for change as modern life changes; and the Reconstructionist Jews follow the culture of the Judaic heritage, but do not believe that Jews are God's chosen people.The Jewish will wash the body, wrap it in a linen shroud, place it in a simple casket and keep the casket closed. They will then wear a torn piece of black cloth to symbolize their grief.

Mormon faith is based on the Book of Mormon. They believe that the souls of the dead can be saved by a living family member that is Mormon. Even if the dead person did not believe in God, a Morman family member will "pray them into heaven".

Orthodox Christians split from the Roman Catholic Church around the year 1000. They adhere to many of the Catholic beliefs, but they reject the jurisdiction of the Pope. They venerate the Virgin Mary.

Protestantism is composed of many different churches. Here, I list them in alphabetical order: The **Baptist** beliefs stem totally from the Bible. They believe in baptism of everyone. The **Church of Christ** members believe in the New Testament. Their baptism is of only adults. **Episcopals** believe in the "Book of Common Prayer" and a modified version of the Bible called the "Thirty Nine Articles". Their baptism is of infants. **Lutherans** believe that salvation comes through faith alone, and infants are baptized. **Methodists** study religion "by rule and method", and study the bible by tradition and reason. They baptize infants and adults. **Pentecostals** speak in tongues and believe in faith healing. They are very boisterious in their sermons and worship. Adults are baptized.

Presbyterianism is based solely on the Bible. The **Seventh Day Adventists** adhere strictly to the Bible with great emphasis on the second coming of Christ. Baptism is reserved for those who are old enough to choose for themselves.

Quakers believe in "The Inner Light" (God's Spirit as it is experienced within each person).They have meetings of quiet meditation without sermon or ritual.

SOME DAY

There's a place that I have dreamed of
The sand slips between your toes
The sun never burns your nose
The wind lightly blows
only happy people go
Let's go there some day!

There's a place I've often thought of
Where the grass is always green
And the air is fresh and clean
Beside a little stream
That no one's ever seen
Let's go there some day

There's a place that I have heard of
Where they have the best of times
And not a soul there ever cries
The atmosphere's divine
Say there'll come a time
To go there some day

There's a place that I've been told of
And you say some day I'll see
Just how wonderfull it will be
When it's time to take me
Heaven is what you mean
Please, God, lead the way

Constance Hope Stringer
2005

Chapter Nine
DOCUMENTS AND DECISIONS

The Living Will

Also Known As "Advanced Directives"

Federal law was passed in 1990 that requires all healthcare agencies to inform all of their patients over the age of 18 that they have the right to accept or refuse treatment, as well as the right to execute an advanced directive. A Living Will is a document stating what you would like done in the event that you stopped breathing, your heart stopped beating, or you are in a coma that the doctors do not believe you will come out of. There are many different circumstances that can not be foreseen, or adequately documented. These things can happen to any of us, at any age, at any time. This is a form, you can have witnessed, that states your general wishes. It is a good idea to discuss different circumstances with a trusted family member or friend so they would be able to state your wishes on your behalf in the event that this form does not cover the circumstances, and you are not able to state them for yourself. Your family should know that you have a Living Will, what it states, and where to find it at all times. You will find a blank Living Will, that I have drafted, in the back of this book.

Show this to your doctor when you are admitted to the hospital and he will convey your wishes by writing the order in your chart.

For some reason, not all Living Wills are legal from state to state. Generally your wishes are followed, and this form makes your wishes very clear. But if you are concerned that there may be a disagreement between your family members or doctors when the time comes, and you want to ensure that your legal rights are honored, consult a lawyer in your state. Some Living Wills are vague. I have seen some that I would never sign, for fear that nothing would be done in the event that I had an easily reversible event. DNR (do not resuscitate) instructions should be followed only under the circumstances that you have outlined. If your religion and/or beliefs dictate that whatever happens is God's will, and that it would be God's will for you to die, it is your choice to make yourself a "DNR", OR A "LIMITED DNR", meaning that there are some things that you do want to be done, and some things that you do not want to be done.

I, personally, believe that God intends for us to take care of ourselves by using any means available. But, I also believe that there are circumstances in which our bodies and minds are beyond repair, and that prolonging that life would only cause more pain and suffering. In this case, I believe, it is time to concentrate on being comfortable, putting any bad feelings we may have behind us, and celebrate the things that make us happy!

1) Initial and date only the sections that apply to you

2) Use a black ink pen for each entry

3) Be sure to have it witnessed

4) Make sure your family knows your wishes

5) You may change your mind at any time. All you have to do is tell your doctor and/or nurse that your wishes have changed!

If you choose not to have a living will, you may want another form of advanced directive called a "durable power of attorney". This is where you name someone to make healthcare decisions on your behalf. You should go to an attorney to have one of these drawn up. This person should know how you feel about things, and you should trust them to make decisions in the event that you become incapacitated.

FINAL ARRANGEMENTS

It is a little known fact that you do not have to make mortuaries rich and you, or your loved ones, broke to be buried. In some states it is legal to be:

1) buried without being embalmed as long as it is done within 24 hours

2) buried in a home-made wooden box

3) buried on your own land

4) have the whole funeral at your own home

Whatever your personal desires for your funeral may be, make your own arrangements before your time comes. If it is a parade you want, set money aside for it. Spare your family the guilt and/or expense. It's your life...your death. You decide, then put it in writing in this book.

Final arrangements involve the care of the body and the ceremonies following a death. The disposition of the body may include a burial (below ground, in a grave), entombment (above ground, in a mausoleum), cremation (burning of the body to bone fragments, usually placed in an urn afterwards. Some religions, such as some Jews, Islams, Orthodox, and a few fundament- alist Chrisians, do not allow cremation.), or donation (to medical science to be used for transplanting useful organs, or learning).

The choice and execution of one of these methods is made with consideration to legal, cultural, and religious requirements. A funeral helps the mourners to come to terms with the death of their loved one. It is usually held from one to four days after the death. Sometimes a memorial service is held that focuses on the life, rather than the death.

Certified copies of death certificates, legal records of a death, are required for death benefits and to settle financial affairs. They may be obtained from the funeral diector for up to six months, after that you must contact the Health Department or Registrar to obtain them. After the terrorists' attack on 9/11 the government made it harder to obtain a death certificate because terrorists were stealing the identities of the deceased. You will need many of them, so speak with the funeral director about how many you will need, get plenty of copies, and keep them in a safe place.

Be A Donor

In 2003 President Bush proclaimed April as "National Donate Life Month". He asked us all to sign organ and tissue donor cards.

Never assume that no part of your body would be acceptable for donation. Even your skin can be a lifesaver to a burn victim. Your state's organ donation center will make that determination when it is contacted by the nurse. Let your family know if you would like to be a donor. You should think about this now. It's your decision. It may also bring comfort to your family to know that a part of your body lives on in another.

In case you are wondering, I choose to have my body donated for whatever parts will help another person have a longer, healthier, happier life. Then the rest is to be donated to science for study (we have to learn some way). This way we all win! I go to heaven, one or more people get needed organs, and my family will not have to pay for my burial. I must add here that my husband has asked that he be given my ashes after they are through with my body, because he wants some part of me to be in the a designated place--my grave--where he can come and "talk" to me. It is important to include the wishes of your loved ones in these arrangements. You see, though it doesn't matter to me what happens to my body when I'm dead, it does matter to my husband and other family members, and that's what matters to me.

God grant me the serenity
To accept the things I can not change
The courage to change
The things I can
And the wisdom
To know the difference

the alcoholic's prayer

THE
MAINTENANCE
LOG

(use colored paper clips to mark frequently used sections)

QUESTIONS AND ANSWERS
Please answer honestly or not at all.

When you think of dying, is pain the first thing you think of, is it your greatest fear?_____

How can you be sure that you will suffer as little pain as possible?_____

Would you rather suffer some pain in order to remain conscious of your surroundings and be aware during the days you have left?_____

At what point would you rather "just go off to sleep" as opposed to remaining in pain?_____

Is death just an eternal slumber, or will you one day "wake up" to another existance?_____

Is there a Heaven and a Hell?_____

Are you afraid to die because you fear the price you will have to pay for your transgressions here on Earth?_____

Could it be that the "worst" of sins require that you spend eternity burning in the hottest of fires while lesser sins will lessen the heat and suffering?_____

If you've been "good" will you go to heaven to live among God?_____

Will there be so may people in Heaven that only the purest of souls will be able to get close enough to see him, let alone talk with him?_____

Will your number and severity of sins determine to what extent you will suffer or rejoyce?_____

What is the worst sin?_____

What sins are unforgiveable?_____

What sins have you committed?_____

What do you have to do to be forgiven of your sins?_____

Must you ask forgiveness of those you have sinned against?

_____

Can you make up for them in any way?_____

Is God your final judge, or are you?_____

If you die feeling guilt-free, will you be?_____

Will you be aware of the lives of those you left behind?_____

Will you even know them?_____

Will you have any memory of your life here on Earth?_____

Will those left here on Earth remember you?_____

What will they remember about you?_____

Will your dying cause a financial burden on others?_____

Who?_____

What could you do to prevent it?_____

Is there something you wish you had said to someone?_____

Done for someone?_____

Do you believe there are those who will mourn for you for reasons other than what you could have done for them?_____

Who?_____

How important is it that others feel that you "died with dignity"?

_____

Do you feel that you would lose some of that respect if you cry, or show anger, or show fear?_____

Who do you feel you could talk openly and honestly to about any of these things?_____

Who do you feel would truely listen?_____

Would you like to be involved with picking-out your own casket, making your own funeral arrangements, or writing your own eulogy?_____

Who do you trust would follow your last wishes ---even if they disagreed?_____

Do you have a durable medical power of attorney?_____

A living will?_____

Do you have a last will and testament?_____

Where are they?_____

Have you ever taken care of someone that was dying?_____

Did you know they were dying?_____

Did they know?_____

Was it a good experience or bad one?_____

Do you feel that you were able to help them in any way?_____

How?_____

Were you afraid you'd do something wrong and do more harm than good?_____
Are you afraid now?_____
What are you most afraid of?_____

PERSONAL INFORMATION

You may circle the ones that apply to you when a choice is given. Leave the line blank if it does not apply to you.

Print Full Name:_____

Place of Birth _____Date of Birth_____

Your Phone Numbers_____

Address_____

Doctor_____ Phone_____

Next of Kin _____

Relationship to you_____

Phone Numbers_____

Hospice?___Phone number_____

Home Health?___Phone Number_____

Alternate Contact _____

Their Phone Numbers_____

Height ____ft. ____ in. Weight _____ Sex_____ Race ___

Primary Language _____

Do You Have a Living Will? _____

Healthcare Power of Attorney?_____Who?_____

Their Phone Numbers _____

Would You Like to be a Donor in the Event of Your

Death? _____ Does Family Know? ___ _____

Do you Smoke? _____How Much? _____

When did you Start? _____Stop? _____

Do You Drink Alcohol Regularly? _____

How Much of What Kind? _____

Do You Have a Drug Problem? _____ What Kind _____

How Much? _____

Do You Wear Glasses/Contacts? _____

Always/ Just for Reading? _____Hard of Hearing? _____

Hearing Aids? _____ Right/Left/Both? _____

Wear Dentures? _____Uppers/Lowers/Both

Chewing Problem? _____ Swallowing? _____

Special Diet? _____

Food Intolerances? _____

Do You Need Anything To Help You Sleep?_____
What?_____

I Have Some Form of Pain Always/ Often/ Never
Where? _____

Why do You Have This Pain? _____

Average Scale? _____What Helps? _____

What Makes it Worse? _____

Do You Have Frequent/Constant Sores? _____

Where? _____ Why? ____ _____

_____

Do You Require Assistance:

To Walk? _____ Turn? _____ Bathe? _____ Eat? _____

Dress? _____

Do You Use:

A Wheelchair? _____ Walker? _____ Cane? _____

Shower Chair?_____Oxygen ___ What Flow?_____

Always/Nights/as Needed?_____

Allergic to Anything? _____ List Them and Their Reaction:

_____

_____

_____

_____

_____

_____

_____

_____

PERSONAL HISTORY

_____

Print full name

Check the left of those you have, or have ever had, then explain to the right.

___ High Blood Pressure_____

___ High Cholesterol _____

___ Stroke_____

___ Fainting/Dizziness_____

___ Heart Failure_____

___ Edema _____

___ Heart Attack _____

___ Heart Surgery _____

___ Heart Catheter_____

___ Cardiac Stress Test_____

___ Implanted Defibrillator _____

___ Pacemaker _____

___ Palpitations _____

___ Arrythmias _____

___ Seizures_____

___ Spinal Cord Injury_____

___ Anemia _____

___ Bleeding Disorder _____

___ Blood Transfusion _____

___ Transfusion Reaction _____

___ Blood Disease_____

___ Hepatitis _____

___ Asthma _____

___ Chronic Bronchitis _____

___ Emphysema_____

___ Tuberculosis_____

___ Thyroid Problems_____

___ Diabetes _____

___ Dialysis _____

___ Fistula/Vas-cath_____

___ Special IV Catheter _____

___ Cancer_____

___ Hiatal Hernia _____

___ Ulcers _____

___ Mental Health Problems _____

___ Other Not Mentioned _____

___ Surgeries List Below:

Date _____ Type _____

Date _____ Type _____

Date _____ Type _____

Date _____ Type _____

Date _____ Type _____

Date _____ Type _____

Date _____ Type _____

Date _____ Type _____

Date _____ Type _____

Date _____ Type _____

Date _____ Type _____

Date _____ Type _____

MY MEDICATIONS

_____

Print full name

Draw a single line through an entry that has been stopped or
changed then make a new entry
The one below is an example only:

Name: ____Lipitor____ # mgs__20__# Tabs _1 _____
times/day __1__times of day _9 pm._____
date stopped_____ date changed _____

Name: _____ # mgs _____ # Tabs _____
times/day _____ times of day _____
date stopped_____ date changed _____

Name: _____ # mgs _____ # Tabs _____
times/day _____ times of day _____
date stopped_____ date changed _____

Name: _____ # mgs _____ # Tabs _____
times/day _____ times of day _____
date stopped_____ date changed _____

Name: _____ # mgs _____ # Tabs _____
times/day _____ times of day _____
date stopped_____ date changed _____

Name: _____ # mgs _____ # Tabs _____
times/day _____ times of day _____
date stopped_____ date changed _____

Name: _____ # mgs _____ # Tabs _____

times/day _____ times of day _____

date stopped_____ date changed _____

Name: _____ # mgs _____ # Tabs _____

times/day _____ times of day _____

date stopped_____ date changed _____

Name: _____ # mgs _____ # Tabs _____

times/day _____ times of day _____

date stopped_____ date changed _____

Name: _____ # mgs _____ # Tabs _____

times/day _____ times of day _____

date stopped_____ date changed _____

Name: _____ # mgs _____ # Tabs _____

times/day _____ times of day _____

date stopped_____ date changed _____

Name: _____ # mgs _____ # Tabs _____

times/day _____ times of day _____

date stopped_____ date changed _____

Name: _____ # mgs _____ # Tabs _____

times/day _____ times of day _____

date stopped_____ date changed _____

Name: _____ # mgs _____ # Tabs _____

times/day _____ times of day _____

date stopped_____ date changed _____

Name: _____ # mgs _____ # Tabs _____

times/day _____ times of day _____

date stopped_____ date changed _____

Name: _____ # mgs _____ # Tabs _____
times/day _____ times of day _____
date stopped_____ date changed _____

Name: _____ # mgs _____ # Tabs _____
times/day _____ times of day _____
date stopped_____ date changed _____

Name: _____ # mgs _____ # Tabs _____
times/day _____ times of day _____
date stopped_____ date changed _____

Name: _____ # mgs _____ # Tabs _____
times/day _____ times of day _____
date stopped_____ date changed _____

Name: _____ # mgs _____ # Tabs _____
times/day _____ times of day _____
date stopped_____ date changed _____

Name: _____ # mgs _____ # Tabs _____
times/day _____ times of day _____
date stopped_____ date changed _____

Name: _____ # mgs _____ # Tabs _____
times/day _____ times of day _____
date stopped_____ date changed _____

Name: _____ # mgs _____ # Tabs _____
times/day _____ times of day _____
date stopped_____ date changed _____

Name: _____ # mgs _____ # Tabs _____
times/day _____ times of day _____
date stopped_____ date changed _____

Name: _____ # mgs _____ # Tabs _____
times/day _____ times of day _____
date stopped_____ date changed _____

Name: _____ # mgs _____ # Tabs _____
times/day _____ times of day _____
date stopped_____ date changed _____

Name: _____ # mgs _____ # Tabs _____
times/day _____ times of day _____
date stopped_____ date changed _____

Name: _____ # mgs _____ # Tabs _____
times/day _____ times of day _____
date stopped_____ date changed _____

Name: _____ # mgs _____ # Tabs _____
times/day _____ times of day _____
date stopped_____ date changed _____

Name: _____ # mgs _____ # Tabs _____
times/day _____ times of day _____
date stopped_____ date changed _____

Name: _____ # mgs _____ # Tabs _____
times/day _____ times of day _____
date stopped_____ date changed _____

Name: _____ # mgs _____ # Tabs _____
times/day _____ times of day _____
date stopped_____ date changed _____

Name: _____ # mgs _____ # Tabs _____
times/day _____ times of day _____
date stopped_____ date changed _____

SPECIAL INSTRUCTIONS FOR MY MEDICINE

_____

Print full name

_____
_____
_____
_____
_____
_____
_____
_____
_____
_____
_____
_____
_____
_____
_____
_____
_____
_____
_____
_____

FREQUENT MEASUREMENTS LOG

_____
Print full name

This card is to be used to log frequent heart rates, blood pressures, blood sugars, or weights

Label _____

Result	Date	Time		Result	Date	Time
_____	_____	_____		_____	_____	_____
_____	_____	_____		_____	_____	_____
_____	_____	_____		_____	_____	_____
_____	_____	_____		_____	_____	_____
_____	_____	_____		_____	_____	_____
_____	_____	_____		_____	_____	_____
_____	_____	_____		_____	_____	_____
_____	_____	_____		_____	_____	_____
_____	_____	_____		_____	_____	_____
_____	_____	_____		_____	_____	_____
_____	_____	_____		_____	_____	_____
_____	_____	_____		_____	_____	_____
_____	_____	_____		_____	_____	_____
_____	_____	_____		_____	_____	_____
_____	_____	_____		_____	_____	_____
_____	_____	_____		_____	_____	_____
_____	_____	_____		_____	_____	_____
_____	_____	_____		_____	_____	_____
_____	_____	_____		_____	_____	_____
_____	_____	_____		_____	_____	_____
_____	_____	_____		_____	_____	_____

Label _____

Result	Date	Time	Result	Date	Time

Label _____

Result	Date	Time	Result	Date	Time

Label _____

Result	Date	Time		Result	Date	Time
------	------	------		------	------	------
------	------	------		------	------	------
------	------	------		------	------	------
------	------	------		------	------	------
------	------	------		------	------	------
------	------	------		------	------	------
------	------	------		------	------	------
------	------	------		------	------	------
------	------	------		------	------	------
------	------	------		------	------	------
------	------	------		------	------	------
------	------	------		------	------	------
------	------	------		------	------	------
------	------	------		------	------	------
------	------	------		------	------	------
------	------	------		------	------	------
------	------	------		------	------	------
------	------	------		------	------	------
------	------	------		------	------	------
------	------	------		------	------	------
------	------	------		------	------	------
------	------	------		------	------	------
------	------	------		------	------	------
------	------	------		------	------	------
------	------	------		------	------	------
------	------	------		------	------	------

DOCTOR OR LABORATORY APPOINTMENTS

_____
Print full name

Date_____ Time _____ Place _____
Result_____

Date_____ Time _____ Place _____
Result_____

Date_____ Time _____ Place _____
Result_____

Date_____ Time _____ Place _____
Result_____

Date_____ Time _____ Place _____
Result_____

Date_____ Time _____ Place _____
Result_____

Date_____ Time _____ Place _____
Result_____

Date_____ Time _____ Place _____
Result_____

Date_____ Time _____ Place _____
Result_____

Date_____ Time _____ Place _____
Result_____

ADMISSIONS TO THE HOSPITAL
OR EMERGENCY DEPARTMENT

_____
Print full name

Date In_____Reason _____
Procedure_____
Doctors_____Date Out_____

Date In_____Reason _____
Procedure_____
Doctors_____Date Out_____

Date In_____Reason _____
Procedure_____
Doctors_____Date Out_____

Date In_____Reason _____
Procedure_____
Doctors_____Date Out_____
Date In_____Reason _____
Procedure_____
Doctors_____Date Out_____

Date In_____Reason _____
Procedure_____
Doctors_____Date Out_____

Date In_____Reason _____
Procedure_____
Doctors_____Date Out_____

Date In_____Reason _____
Procedure_____
Doctors_____Date Out_____

FUNERAL AND BURIAL INSTRUCTIONS

Print Full Name_____

_____
_____
_____
_____
_____
_____
_____
_____
_____
_____
_____
_____
_____
_____
_____
_____
_____
_____
_____
_____
_____
_____
_____
_____
_____
_____

NOTES

NOTES

NOTES

NOTES

_____
_____
_____
_____
_____
_____
_____
_____
_____
_____
_____
_____
_____
_____
_____
_____
_____
_____
_____
_____
_____
_____
_____
_____
_____
_____
_____
_____
_____

THE LIVING WILL OF

_____
Print full name

In the event of a **terminal illness** or **vegetive state** I am to be treated, medically and personally, as anyone else with the exception of the items specifically listed below:

1) It is my will that I not be resusitated under any circumstances. Initials_____Date_____

2) I have a terminal illness that my doctor calls: _____
Initials_____Date_____

3) It is my will to be made comfortable with whatever medications and dosages my doctors have ordered for me, without concideration to the effects it may have on my level of consciousness. Initials _____ Date _____

4) It is my will that I take food and fluids only when I am able and willing to partake of them myself, and at no time is anyone to force them upon me, directly or indirectly.
Initials _____ Date _____

5) It is my will that I not be intubated (breathing tube placed in the lungs) under any circumstances. Initials _____
Date _____

6) It is my will that I not be placed on a ventilator (breathing machine).Initials _____ Date _____

7) It is my will that I not be defibrillated (have my heart shocked). Initials _____ Date _____

8) It is my will that my remains be cremated (burned). Initials _____ Date _____

9) It is my will that my remains be donated to science (for study). Initials _____ Date _____

10) It is my will that part of my body be donated (for transplant into a living body).
Initials _____ Date _____

Print Name_____

Signature _____Date_____

Address_____

Phone Number_____

Witness #1:

Print Name_____

Signature_____Date _____

Address_____

Phone Number_____

Relationship_____

Witness #2:

Print Name_____

Signature_____Date _____

Address_____

Phone Number_____

Relationship_____

Witness of someone NOT related to you, that will not benefit from your death:

Print Name_____

Signature_____Date _____

Address_____

Phone Number_____

PAIN MEDICATIONS ADMINISTERED

Date:____Time:____Med:_____Amount:_____
Date:____Time:____Med:_____Amount:_____
Date:____Time:____Med:_____Amount:_____
Date:____Time:____Med:_____Amount:_____
Date:____Time:____Med:_____Amount:_____
Date:____Time:____Med:_____Amount:_____
Date:____Time:____Med:_____Amount:_____
Date:____Time:____Med:_____Amount:_____
Date:____Time:____Med:_____Amount:_____
Date:____Time:____Med:_____Amount:_____
Date:____Time:____Med:_____Amount:_____
Date:____Time:____Med:_____Amount:_____
Date:____Time:____Med:_____Amount:_____
Date:____Time:____Med:_____Amount:_____
Date:____Time:____Med:_____Amount:_____
Date:____Time:____Med:_____Amount:_____
Date:____Time:____Med:_____Amount:_____
Date:____Time:____Med:_____Amount:_____
Date:____Time:____Med:_____Amount:_____
Date:____Time:____Med:_____Amount:_____
Date:____Time:____Med:_____Amount:_____
Date:____Time:____Med:_____Amount:_____
Date:____Time:____Med:_____Amount:_____
Date:____Time:____Med:_____Amount:_____
Date:____Time:____Med:_____Amount:_____
Date:____Time:____Med:_____Amount:_____
Date:____Time:____Med:_____Amount:_____
Date:____Time:____Med:_____Amount:_____
Date:____Time:____Med:_____Amount:_____
Date:____Time:____Med:_____Amount:_____
Date:____Time:____Med:_____Amount:_____
Date:____Time:____Med:_____Amount:_____
Date:____Time:____Med:_____Amount:_____
Date:____Time:____Med:_____Amount:_____
Date:____Time:____Med:_____Amount:_____

PAIN MEDICATIONS ADMINISTERED

Date:____Time:____Med:_____Amount:_____
Date:____Time:____Med:_____Amount:_____
Date:____Time:____Med:_____Amount:_____
Date:____Time:____Med:_____Amount:_____
Date:____Time:____Med:_____Amount:_____
Date:____Time:____Med:_____Amount:_____
Date:____Time:____Med:_____Amount:_____
Date:____Time:____Med:_____Amount:_____
Date:____Time:____Med:_____Amount:_____
Date:____Time:____Med:_____Amount:_____
Date:____Time:____Med:_____Amount:_____
Date:____Time:____Med:_____Amount:_____
Date:____Time:____Med:_____Amount:_____
Date:____Time:____Med:_____Amount:_____
Date:____Time:____Med:_____Amount:_____
Date:____Time:____Med:_____Amount:_____
Date:____Time:____Med:_____Amount:_____
Date:____Time:____Med:_____Amount:_____
Date:____Time:____Med:_____Amount:_____
Date:____Time:____Med:_____Amount:_____
Date:____Time:____Med:_____Amount:_____
Date:____Time:____Med:_____Amount:_____
Date:____Time:____Med:_____Amount:_____
Date:____Time:____Med:_____Amount:_____
Date:____Time:____Med:_____Amount:_____
Date:____Time:____Med:_____Amount:_____
Date:____Time:____Med:_____Amount:_____
Date:____Time:____Med:_____Amount:_____
Date:____Time:____Med:_____Amount:_____
Date:____Time:____Med:_____Amount:_____
Date:____Time:____Med:_____Amount:_____
Date:____Time:____Med:_____Amount:_____
Date:____Time:____Med:_____Amount:_____
Date:____Time:____Med:_____Amount:_____
Date:____Time:____Med:_____Amount:_____

PAIN MEDICATIONS ADMINISTERED

Date:____Time:____Med:_____Amount:_____
Date:____Time:____Med:_____Amount:_____
Date:____Time:____Med:_____Amount:_____
Date:____Time:____Med:_____Amount:_____
Date:____Time:____Med:_____Amount:_____
Date:____Time:____Med:_____Amount:_____
Date:____Time:____Med:_____Amount:_____
Date:____Time:____Med:_____Amount:_____
Date:____Time:____Med:_____Amount:_____
Date:____Time:____Med:_____Amount:_____
Date:____Time:____Med:_____Amount:_____
Date:____Time:____Med:_____Amount:_____
Date:____Time:____Med:_____Amount:_____
Date:____Time:____Med:_____Amount:_____
Date:____Time:____Med:_____Amount:_____
Date:____Time:____Med:_____Amount:_____
Date:____Time:____Med:_____Amount:_____
Date:____Time:____Med:_____Amount:_____
Date:____Time:____Med:_____Amount:_____
Date:____Time:____Med:_____Amount:_____
Date:____Time:____Med:_____Amount:_____
Date:____Time:____Med:_____Amount:_____
Date:____Time:____Med:_____Amount:_____
Date:____Time:____Med:_____Amount:_____
Date:____Time:____Med:_____Amount:_____
Date:____Time:____Med:_____Amount:_____
Date:____Time:____Med:_____Amount:_____
Date:____Time:____Med:_____Amount:_____
Date:____Time:____Med:_____Amount:_____
Date:____Time:____Med:_____Amount:_____
Date:____Time:____Med:_____Amount:_____
Date:____Time:____Med:_____Amount:_____
Date:____Time:____Med:_____Amount:_____
Date:____Time:____Med:_____Amount:_____
Date:____Time:____Med:_____Amount:_____

PAIN MEDICATIONS ADMINISTERED

Date:___Time:___Med:_____Amount:_____
Date:___Time:___Med:_____Amount:_____
Date:___Time:___Med:_____Amount:_____
Date:___Time:___Med:_____Amount:_____
Date:___Time:___Med:_____Amount:_____
Date:___Time:___Med:_____Amount:_____
Date:___Time:___Med:_____Amount:_____
Date:___Time:___Med:_____Amount:_____
Date:___Time:___Med:_____Amount:_____
Date:___Time:___Med:_____Amount:_____
Date:___Time:___Med:_____Amount:_____
Date:___Time:___Med:_____Amount:_____
Date:___Time:___Med:_____Amount:_____
Date:___Time:___Med:_____Amount:_____
Date:___Time:___Med:_____Amount:_____
Date:___Time:___Med:_____Amount:_____
Date:___Time:___Med:_____Amount:_____
Date:___Time:___Med:_____Amount:_____
Date:___Time:___Med:_____Amount:_____
Date:___Time:___Med:_____Amount:_____
Date:___Time:___Med:_____Amount:_____
Date:___Time:___Med:_____Amount:_____
Date:___Time:___Med:_____Amount:_____
Date:___Time:___Med:_____Amount:_____
Date:___Time:___Med:_____Amount:_____
Date:___Time:___Med:_____Amount:_____
Date:___Time:___Med:_____Amount:_____
Date:___Time:___Med:_____Amount:_____
Date:___Time:___Med:_____Amount:_____
Date:___Time:___Med:_____Amount:_____
Date:___Time:___Med:_____Amount:_____
Date:___Time:___Med:_____Amount:_____
Date:___Time:___Med:_____Amount:_____
Date:___Time:___Med:_____Amount:_____

PAIN MEDICATIONS ADMINISTERED

Date:____Time:____Med:_____Amount:_____
Date:____Time:____Med:_____Amount:_____
Date:____Time:____Med:_____Amount:_____
Date:____Time:____Med:_____Amount:_____
Date:____Time:____Med:_____Amount:_____
Date:____Time:____Med:_____Amount:_____
Date:____Time:____Med:_____Amount:_____
Date:____Time:____Med:_____Amount:_____
Date:____Time:____Med:_____Amount:_____
Date:____Time:____Med:_____Amount:_____
Date:____Time:____Med:_____Amount:_____
Date:____Time:____Med:_____Amount:_____
Date:____Time:____Med:_____Amount:_____
Date:____Time:____Med:_____Amount:_____
Date:____Time:____Med:_____Amount:_____
Date:____Time:____Med:_____Amount:_____
Date:____Time:____Med:_____Amount:_____
Date:____Time:____Med:_____Amount:_____
Date:____Time:____Med:_____Amount:_____
Date:____Time:____Med:_____Amount:_____
Date:____Time:____Med:_____Amount:_____
Date:____Time:____Med:_____Amount:_____
Date:____Time:____Med:_____Amount:_____
Date:____Time:____Med:_____Amount:_____
Date:____Time:____Med:_____Amount:_____
Date:____Time:____Med:_____Amount:_____
Date:____Time:____Med:_____Amount:_____
Date:____Time:____Med:_____Amount:_____
Date:____Time:____Med:_____Amount:_____
Date:____Time:____Med:_____Amount:_____
Date:____Time:____Med:_____Amount:_____
Date:____Time:____Med:_____Amount:_____
Date:____Time:____Med:_____Amount:_____
Date:____Time:____Med:_____Amount:_____

PAIN MEDICATIONS ADMINISTERED

Date:____Time:____Med:_____Amount:_____
Date:____Time:____Med:_____Amount:_____
Date:____Time:____Med:_____Amount:_____
Date:____Time:____Med:_____Amount:_____
Date:____Time:____Med:_____Amount:_____
Date:____Time:____Med:_____Amount:_____
Date:____Time:____Med:_____Amount:_____
Date:____Time:____Med:_____Amount:_____
Date:____Time:____Med:_____Amount:_____
Date:____Time:____Med:_____Amount:_____
Date:____Time:____Med:_____Amount:_____
Date:____Time:____Med:_____Amount:_____
Date:____Time:____Med:_____Amount:_____
Date:____Time:____Med:_____Amount:_____
Date:____Time:____Med:_____Amount:_____
Date:____Time:____Med:_____Amount:_____
Date:____Time:____Med:_____Amount:_____
Date:____Time:____Med:_____Amount:_____
Date:____Time:____Med:_____Amount:_____
Date:____Time:____Med:_____Amount:_____
Date:____Time:____Med:_____Amount:_____
Date:____Time:____Med:_____Amount:_____
Date:____Time:____Med:_____Amount:_____
Date:____Time:____Med:_____Amount:_____
Date:____Time:____Med:_____Amount:_____
Date:____Time:____Med:_____Amount:_____
Date:____Time:____Med:_____Amount:_____
Date:____Time:____Med:_____Amount:_____
Date:____Time:____Med:_____Amount:_____
Date:____Time:____Med:_____Amount:_____
Date:____Time:____Med:_____Amount:_____
Date:____Time:____Med:_____Amount:_____
Date:____Time:____Med:_____Amount:_____
Date:____Time:____Med:_____Amount:_____

DAILY ACTIVITY LOG
AND NOTES TO CAREGIVERS

DAILY ACTIVITY LOG
AND NOTES TO CAREGIVERS

DAILY ACTIVITY LOG
AND NOTES TO CAREGIVERS

DAILY ACTIVITY LOG
AND NOTES TO CAREGIVERS

_____
_____
_____
_____
_____
_____
_____
_____
_____
_____
_____
_____
_____
_____
_____
_____
_____
_____
_____
_____
_____
_____
_____
_____
_____
_____
_____
_____
_____

DAILY ACTIVITY LOG
AND NOTES TO CAREGIVERS

_____
_____
_____
_____
_____
_____
_____
_____
_____
_____
_____
_____
_____
_____
_____
_____
_____
_____
_____
_____
_____
_____
_____
_____
_____
_____
_____
_____

DAILY ACTIVITY LOG
AND NOTES TO CAREGIVERS

DAILY ACTIVITY LOG
AND NOTES TO CAREGIVERS

_____
_____
_____
_____
_____
_____
_____
_____
_____
_____
_____
_____
_____
_____
_____
_____
_____
_____
_____
_____
_____
_____
_____
_____
_____
_____
_____
_____
_____

DAILY ACTIVITY LOG
AND NOTES TO CAREGIVERS

DAILY ACTIVITY LOG
AND NOTES TO CAREGIVERS

_____
_____
_____
_____
_____
_____
_____
_____
_____
_____
_____
_____
_____
_____
_____
_____
_____
_____
_____
_____
_____
_____
_____
_____
_____
_____
_____
_____
_____
_____

DAILY ACTIVITY LOG
AND NOTES TO CAREGIVERS

DAILY ACTIVITY LOG
AND NOTES TO CAREGIVERS

_____
_____
_____
_____
_____
_____
_____
_____
_____
_____
_____
_____
_____
_____
_____
_____
_____
_____
_____
_____
_____
_____
_____
_____
_____
_____
_____

DAILY ACTIVITY LOG
AND NOTES TO CAREGIVERS

_____
_____
_____
_____
_____
_____
_____
_____
_____
_____
_____
_____
_____
_____
_____
_____
_____
_____
_____
_____
_____
_____
_____
_____
_____
_____
_____
_____
_____

DAILY ACTIVITY LOG
AND NOTES TO CAREGIVERS

DAILY ACTIVITY LOG
AND NOTES TO CAREGIVERS

DAILY ACTIVITY LOG
AND NOTES TO CAREGIVERS

_____
_____
_____
_____
_____
_____
_____
_____
_____
_____
_____
_____
_____
_____
_____
_____
_____
_____
_____
_____
_____
_____
_____
_____
_____
_____
_____
_____
_____
_____

DAILY ACTIVITY LOG
AND NOTES TO CAREGIVERS

DAILY ACTIVITY LOG
AND NOTES TO CAREGIVERS

_____
_____
_____
_____
_____
_____
_____
_____
_____
_____
_____
_____
_____
_____
_____
_____
_____
_____
_____
_____
_____
_____
_____
_____
_____
_____
_____
_____

DAILY ACTIVITY LOG
AND NOTES TO CAREGIVERS

DAILY ACTIVITY LOG
AND NOTES TO CAREGIVERS

DAILY ACTIVITY LOG
AND NOTES TO CAREGIVERS

DAILY ACTIVITY LOG
AND NOTES TO CAREGIVERS

DAILY ACTIVITY LOG
AND NOTES TO CAREGIVERS

_____
_____
_____
_____
_____
_____
_____
_____
_____
_____
_____
_____
_____
_____
_____
_____
_____
_____
_____
_____
_____
_____
_____
_____
_____
_____
_____
_____

DAILY ACTIVITY LOG
AND NOTES TO CAREGIVERS

_____
_____
_____
_____
_____
_____
_____
_____
_____
_____
_____
_____
_____
_____
_____
_____
_____
_____
_____
_____
_____
_____
_____
_____
_____
_____
_____
_____
_____
_____
_____

DAILY ACTIVITY LOG
AND NOTES TO CAREGIVERS

DAILY ACTIVITY LOG
AND NOTES TO CAREGIVERS

DAILY ACTIVITY LOG
AND NOTES TO CAREGIVERS

STILL ALIVE

I'M SORRY FOR YOUR LOSS
I DO KNOW HOW YOU FEEL
I LOST MY PARTNER YEARS AGO
AND THE PAIN IS STILL SO REAL

I HAVE LEARNED TO LOVE ANOTHER
HE KNOWS WHAT I'VE BEEN THROUGH
MY PAIN ALMOST CONSUMED ME
BUT MY LOVE FOR HIM IS TRUE

THOUGH I STILL LOVE ANOTHER
HE'S GONE TO LIVE WITH GOD
IT HAPPENED MANY YEARS AGO
AND I STILL SPEAK OF HIM ALOT

I NEVER HAVE TO HIDE IT
MY HUSBAND UNDERSTANDS
AND HE IS NEVER JEALOUS
OF MY LOVE FOR THIS OTHER MAN

THERE WAS A TIME I BELIEVED
I COULD BE NO OTHERS' WIFE
THAT I COULD NEVER FEEL
THIS HAPPY TO BE ALIVE

I WANTED TO DIE WITH ERNIE
I FELT GUILTY FOR SO MUCH
NOW I LOVE MY HUSBAND, GLENN
AND THANK GOD FOR HIS LOVE

Constance Hope Stringer
2005

Answer To The Riddle

NOTHING!

More About Hospice

When a person who qualifies elects to enter the Hospice program they will sign an election form stating that they understand that the care is palliative: for pain relief and symptom control, not curative therapy. Hospices do nothing to speed up or slow down the dying process.

If a person makes the decision to join Hospice, and later feels that they are recovering from their illness, they may elect to be discharged so that they can return to aggressive therapy. If the treatments fail, Medicare, and most private insurance, will allow for coverage should they elect to return to Hospice.

Though Hospice believes that physical, emotional, and spiritual support is needed to treat "the whole person", it does not require its' patients to hold any particular beliefs in relation to religion.

Some Hospices require a small co-payment for medications or respite care. Respite care is where someone stays with the patient, or they are admitted to the hospital for a short time, in order to allow the family and/or caregivers time away. Ask your Hospice provider what their requirements are.

Hospice care is provided by Medicare nationwide and by Medicaid in most states. It is also an option with most private insurance companies. See the websites listed below for specific information on Hospice programs near you.

1) To answer other questions you may have about hospice go to the web at www.hospiceweb.com/faq.htm.

2) For information on Hospice, how to become a volunteer or how to make a donation go the wedsite for the *International Association For Hospice & Palliative Care* at http://www. hospicecare.com/

3) For a state-specific Advanced Directive go to www. consumers@nhpco.org

ABOUT THE AUTHOR

Mrs Stringer continues to work as a Registered Nurse while she writes. She and her husband, Glenn, have recently moved to Kentucky to be near family and friends that are dear to her.

She dedicates this book to her youngest sister, Elana Amos (who's been more like an older sister), and her dearest friend Dolly Chester... **The Three Musketeers; one for all and all for one....Forever!**

www.ingramcontent.com/pod-product-compliance
Lightning Source LLC
Chambersburg PA
CBHW020439290526
45785CB00002B/923